Contents

CW01501117

Nothing
for Granted

by

K.M. Weber

Published by New Generation Publishing in 2024

ISBN: 9781835634714

New Generation Publishing
www.newgeneration-publishing.com

FOREWORD

Thump, thump, thump. I swiftly took large strides in my practical block heels as I dashed from my bus towards the underground station. I noticed my new knee-length coat was floating nicely as I walked: a lovely purchase. The pavement under the bridge stank of urine and I wished I already had my daily commute behind me. Thump, thump, thump. I hoped I would at least catch my first train home. Then I noticed her, a slender woman in her 20s screaming her sorrow and anger out, with a London accent. She jumped bizarrely, throwing her arms in the air as she cursed. I was startled as I recognised myself in her. I too had once been as vulnerable and alienated as she appeared to be.

My personal journey indeed had been from being one of the "regular people" as I would call them, to being an ill person shouting in the street. I had become a mental health patient rather unexpectedly in my thirties, but fortunately I had bounced back, perhaps also unexpectedly. And now I was back to being that busy commuter again.

You do not need to have a prior condition in order to experience poor health, and you do not necessarily have to remain unwell afterward. Things can come and go. Life is transient and nothing is for granted.

Joining the crowd at the entrance to the station I left her behind, but I now dedicate my memoir to that woman I saw in this crowded big city street in 2021. I hope she, or someone similar, can benefit one day from my writing.

CHAPTER ONE – THE REPORTER

"Help! Mummy, help!" a child's shriek pierced the morning quiet like a tiny stone shot with a catapult. Bright light flooded my bedsit despite the faded green curtains drawn over my three large sash windows. All my windows overlooked the pavement, and every sound from the street echoed in my room. The squeaky cries for help came from the street.

Having lain awake for most of the night, I jumped out of my bed. Pulling my only working window frame up as much as it allowed, I stuck my head out. The early morning air was fresh and cool. There were no pedestrians in Harlesden Gardens yet. Among the vehicles parallel parked along my side of the street, one car had its passenger door wide open. A fox was prancing in front of the open door. The child seemed to be strapped in the car, alone and terrified of the animal. I knew I was too far away to help if the fox were to attack this little person.

"Ah, this is our fox!" I shouted out into the air with the hope of at least calming down the owner of the high-pitched voice. The child went quiet, although I was not certain whether my voice had been calming or perhaps even more distressing to them, or if I had been heard at all. The fox disappeared from my view.

"I am here baby, I'm back." A woman came out of the front door two houses away from me, trying to soothe her child.

I pulled my head back into my room. That was me ready for the day. My jogging suit I had worn at night did not require changing. My messy straw-like hair did not require tidying up. My teeth did not require immediate cleaning, and there was no shower anytime soon in my plans. My day had no purpose. I had nothing to look forward to, no commitments to keep, and no friends to meet. I was going through my mental breakdown, and I looked a mess. I would only need to eat something later, and, if there was no food left at my place, I might venture out to the nearby cashpoint and then to some food stores in the area. I might visit specific stores for some groceries that I felt were more magical than others – perhaps to buy some more of those large round flat tins of Brazilian banana jam that I thought could serve as the wheels my life needed to move on far from where I was parked in 2009.

***

Harlesden, a former village that is now part of North-west London, was a good place for buying international food. There was a Caribbean bakery near Harlesden's main landmark, the 19th-century free-standing Jubilee Clock. I sometimes liked to walk over and try their products, some of which were a novelty for me. I usually chose their cinnamon buns, or slices of different loaf cakes, like Madeira cake, rum cake, or bread pudding. They also served some hot savoury patties, very spicy ones. The bakery was under-explored by the non-Caribbean locals, and I was normally the only pale person in the queue. Two streets across from the Caribbean bakery, also near Jubilee Clock's little junction, there was a rice and meat takeaway run by some Pakistani staff, and I also sometimes bought their tasty food in their little square Styrofoam boxes. Some of those boxes with bits of leftover meat and bones were dropped by careless customers in the streets around, a feast for animals overnight.

There were some Caribbean takeaways, one of which served some delicious carrot drinks with some spices and a dash of milk. There were also some Brazilian restaurants and a Brazilian supermarket. The small businesses in the area mostly had customers from their own geographical backgrounds. The local Middle Eastern supermarket sold a lot of Asian and East-European food. There were, however, no English restaurants on this patch of England. As someone who had chosen England for my home, I wished there were.

The Somali owner of my local internet café round the corner from Harlesden Gardens greeted me in his friendly manner, "Hello Zainab, how are you today?"

My name is not Zainab. However, I liked this nickname he had invented for me. It is a Muslim female name that must have reminded him of his home and of everything that mattered to him. I appreciated that.

His name was Ghaazi, or Ghais; his was one of two or three Somali-owned internet access and phone repair shops near the free-standing clock. Ghais wore his traditional white robe and a white kufi cap, and he would greet me even outside his shop. I was one of his regular customers.

I was 36 at the time, and my NHS doctor in Harlesden's mental health centre had told me I was probably never going to be fit for work again, which sounded disastrous to me. I had no family of my own, so my jobs had been my all. I dreamt of doing something meaningful. I had brought my various hand-written notes with me to get them scanned at Ghais's shop. Then I posted my scanned scrawlings online. I meant to write about what was wrong with the world. I saw myself as a kind of a reporter, although my notes were made of scrambled words and phrases that made no sense to the reader. I was going through psychosis, and my thinking process was largely distorted. I was a reporter from the other side of madness.

"Zainab, what you need is a lot of sleep. You are having a problem, and you need some really good rest," Ghais would say.

***

I am not entirely sure why I developed psychosis, but I have a feeling it may have been related to my life-long obsession of always having to deliver. I probably loved myself too little, so any criticism I ever received was amplified many times over in my mind, echoing over and over. I am a Polish woman by birth, and I used to be a professional before I ended up buying my magical tins of food during my 2009 psychosis.

Having spent six years in higher education, I had become a Sworn Translator of English Language in my native Poland at the age of 25. I had considered myself a success at the time. I had translated people's documents, stamping my official seal on the paperwork I produced. "Sworn" meant I had initially had to take an oath in my local court of law that I would translate to the best of my knowledge and ability. I had received a round metal seal made by my country's mint with my name on it, and I had had my work periodically reviewed by the court.

Interestingly, I had not earned much from that job. Those days, in Poland, the price of sworn translation had been fixed by an act of parliament instructing us to charge "not more than" a certain percentage of the country's average salary. Formal sworn translations had effectively been made cheaper than other, non-certified translations with a free market price. I had provided inexpensive services for the benefit of the public for the prestige of it, on top of my day job as a schoolteacher.

Before I had been appointed Sworn Translator in 1998, the local police had made checks on me. My clear criminal check had not sufficed. The police had visited my family home, and they had even visited some of my neighbours to enquire about my character. I had apparently passed their screening, as my neighbours had only had good things to say about me. I then always felt that I had to keep my life and all my affairs crystal clean. I felt as though the world needed me flawless, and I expected nothing less of myself. That perfectionist attitude may have contributed to the acuteness of my anxiety a decade later. You should be more generous to yourself than I had been being to myself.

Translating is a never-ending adventure. In the first months of my work, I was contacted by a Polish factory that needed me for their international shareholder meeting.

"We need a sworn translator for our voting procedure," they said, "It is a formality. You will only have to say in English what the voting results are, and we will need your invoice for our records. Everything has already been translated into English and all the foreign shareholders will have their own interpreters, so there will not be much for you to do."

I requested some materials from the factory so that I could familiarise myself with their specialised vocabulary. Unfortunately, they only sent me a fax with a few large hand-written words, 'FOR, AGAINST, ABSTAINED.'

I arrived at their meeting wearing a string of my tiny colourful hippie beads with my otherwise smart suit. I never felt I belonged with the uniformed corporate crowd entirely, and the tiny beads were my lucky charm. Their conference room was full of people. I was greeted with a professional handshake and a few welcoming words by a couple of the factory representatives. Then one of them walked over to me again.

"Our English shareholder has arrived with no interpreter," he said, "Would you mind interpreting for him during our meeting?"

I tried my best. Seated beside him, I whispered along to the English shareholder while somebody was reading out their report to the microphone. You must be very focused for this type of interpreting. You listen to somebody and at the same time you whisper your translation of what they have said a few seconds earlier. It was my first ever simultaneous interpreting assignment, and it had come as a surprise. The speaker's vocabulary became more technical, which was difficult for me, and I felt more and more desperate. The room was in the basement. I fixed my eyes on the fire escape ladder leading up to a window at the top of the wall. I wished I could climb up that ladder and escape through the window.

"He is now talking about different kinds of engines. Kill me but I have no idea how to translate it," I whispered to my English client in the end, without turning to him, my eyes on the speaker.

The English shareholder looked at me stunned, then he also turned back toward the speaker.

"Don't worry at all," he whispered back to me, motionless, "They had emailed me the translation of all this text in advance. I don't even know why they had you interpret this during the meeting for me. How old are you? You look very young."

"No, I am already 25," I whispered back.

"Still very young," his whisper was, "Translating must be a very difficult job."

He was not old himself. We spent the rest of the meeting looking ahead while chatting quietly under our breaths. He told me jokes to put me at ease. I could not laugh, but I could not help smiling and I felt my seat beside him was the best place to be.

"Thank you very much," grinned the factory representatives to me later, "You did wonderfully."

"My" shareholder had clearly not given the game away.

CHAPTER TWO – THE NEWCOMER

I came to the UK from Poland on my student visa in 2003. I came alone. I may have been an English teacher and translator in my native country, but I had only learned from my course books without going abroad, and I felt my English was artificial. I had not been fluent enough to navigate all varieties of the spoken language. However, when I first set my foot on British soil, English was ringing out all around me and that kept my spirits high.

The Caledonian Road Hostel in Islington, with its rows of £75-a-week bunk beds, was home to a variety of guests from different continents. Among the young women in my dormitory room, there was also a local English girl who worked as a teacher but seemed to prefer living in that international commune long-term rather than renting a more traditional home. There was a group of Polish university students who I heard muttering in the kitchen about whether the English genuinely liked orange marmalade so much, or if they always gave us marmalade for breakfast through spite.

Indeed, the hostel management always supplied us with white bread and butter with marmalade for breakfast, along with some cereals and milk, and tea and coffee. This daily breakfast was included in the hostel's weekly accommodation price. There was a social room downstairs where you could meet guests from outside your dorm room. I met some Ugandan male students there, one of whom had 27 brothers and sisters from his father's many wives. He and I spent one

Sunday together, sightseeing, and chatting, which is how I knew about his family and about his siblings. We even went to church to a Sunday service together.

"It says here, Pentecostal. That is not my church, I am Catholic," I said at first.

"Oh, come on. If it says it's a church, I know it is a church. We are going in," he said. And we did.

2003 was one year before my native Poland joined the European Union, which the United Kingdom was part of, so there was not yet free movement between the two countries, and applying for a visa was a natural part of my migration process. I enrolled in an English language school in Holloway Road, North London, and started looking for a job. My student visa, stamped in my passport at border control in Dover, stated that I was allowed part-time employment in the United Kingdom for the whole six months of my permitted stay.

July was a hot, dry month in London, which was convenient for me as I tried to get everywhere on foot. I didn't want to spend any money on public transport before securing myself a job, so I relentlessly trod London pavements. I stepped into cafés, hotels and restaurants to enquire about possible vacancies, always hearing no for an answer. Meanwhile my feet in sandals were getting ruined from the dust in the hot summer streets full of never-ending traffic.

"Hey, slim!" I heard a male voice say one day above my head near my hostel.

The buildings near the hostel in Caledonian Road were covered with bright sunny patches and I had to squint my eyes to look up. Three men wearing enormous colourful woolly hats were smoking in an open window.

"Slim!" repeated one.

I looked around. The street nearby was empty, so Slim had to be me. I had been warned in my new hostel that the streets near Kings Cross area were "rough and full of sex workers", so I walked away briskly though.

Since my teenage years, I had always compared myself

against various beauty standards I had ever read about. That is how I knew I was *not* a beauty. Some magazines for women advised on attractive facial proportions and, although my chin, forehead, and the distance between my eyes seemed correct, my nose was too prominent, and my eyebrows asymmetric. Judging by standard clothing sizes, my chest seemed too small when compared to my hips. My thighs seemed too large. The only part of me that seemed precisely correct was my waist.

Some magazines said Marilyn Monroe had had a waist to hips ratio of 0.7, which had apparently been considered a modern standard for female beauty. Whatever her waist had been, my waist-to-hips ratio was also 0.7 and I had been happy and proud to match at least one printed beauty standard. When I was called Slim in the street just before my 30th birthday, I felt partially relieved that my 0.7 ratio waist may have been more visible from a distance than my plain face. I was made of ratios, measurements, and gradients, and I was still in the process of learning to like my own looks.

I stepped into a small hotel in Kingsland Road in Hackney, London.

"Excuse me, do you need any help?" I asked in my plain English.

"No, we don't," said the man at the reception.

"That's okay, thank you," I smiled turning to the door.

"Wait," the man said, "Why don't you leave your phone number, and I'll call you when we have a vacancy for you."

"Oh, my number... I only have my Polish mobile."

"That's not a problem, I can phone your Polish number. That is, when something comes up."

How poorly equipped I was for life abroad. I did leave my number, although I never expected to be called back.

One Afrikaner girl at my hostel, after two months of looking for work, started sleeping her days through on the bunk bed next to mine. I tried to be active, and I kept on walking around. I found a vacancy clearing tables that was being advertised at our local Job Centre.

"Do you have experience clearing tables at a school canteen?" asked me the Job Centre advisor.

"No, but I have worked at a school. I worked in Polish schools as a teacher."

"Unfortunately, for this position you would need to have at least four years' experience clearing tables."

I envied the street sweepers I regularly passed by. I felt I should be able to sweep, too, although I did not know where to apply. I considered walking up to one of the men to ask how he had managed to get this job. I never did though. I did not want him to feel I was being sarcastic.

Reading a noticeboard in front of one Catholic Church, I saw the address of a day centre for the homeless. I walked to the centre and asked to speak to Becky, the Volunteer Coordinator, whose name I remembered from the church noticeboard. She invited me for a chat.

"We still need to talk about equal opportunities," she said finally. "Our users and volunteers are from all backgrounds and all walks of life. I need to make sure you understand everybody deserves equal opportunities, regardless of their race or background."

"Oh, I am very open to people of all races and backgrounds. I have friends of all races."

"No, it is not about what friends you have. I also could say I have friends of all races, but this is not what it is about."

"Of course, I understand everybody should be given best opportunities, no matter what their ethnicity or background."

"That's still not it," sighed Becky, "but I will write down we have talked about equal opportunities."

I was accepted as a volunteer there. I cannot overstate how much this meant to me. After getting turned down everywhere else, I suddenly managed to get an unpaid job. I met other people at the centre, and I felt a priceless sense of purpose. It did not matter that there was no money on offer. I felt I was being given a chance.

The centre offered shower facilities, a change of clothes, a hot drink, sandwiches, and some fruit. No hot food was being served at the time. There were some religious people among the volunteers, including some nuns. Some other volunteers were unemployed and trying to get references for their job search. One of the volunteers told me she was there because the day centre refunded public transport tickets, so whenever she wanted to travel across London, she popped in. There were also some corporate employees on their volunteering day.

"I am not sure what I should be doing, as much as I would love to be useful," said one bank employee to his colleague on their volunteering day. "Ah, Chris is pouring tea, how on earth did he land that job?"

One other male volunteer told a centre user he should not be there scrounging for food. The user got very upset.

"I have a right to be here!" he shouted, "I am a rough sleeper!"

Grace, a black lady with an accent I thought was West Indian, came out of the kitchen with a tea towel in her hand and stood between the two men.

"Talk to me," she said to the centre user, "What happened?"

The rough sleeper started complaining to Grace, then he remembered the male volunteer and turned back to him, tugging aggressively at his clothes. The atmosphere in the room got tense, there was a fight brewing up. The upset rough sleeper pushed the guilty male volunteer. The men around stepped closer in case they needed to intervene. Grace fearlessly stood between the two agitated men with her tea towel still in her hands. She was determined not to lose the rough sleeper's attention.

"Look at me! You are talking to me, not to him. You are talking to me!"

The upset rough sleeper's anger evaporated as he looked at her.

"Love you, Grace", he finally said to her as he stepped aside.

"Love you too," she smiled and went back to the kitchen.

"Can you come along with me?" one supervisor said to

the volunteer, and as she walked away with him, everyone relaxed.

I was placed near the kitchen area, where I poured tea, distributed sandwiches, sometimes helped washing up, and cleared the tables. Talking to the centre users was a big part of the job. There was a nice young rough-sleeping Englishman called Rhys, his cheeky Jamaican friend Terry, who asked me whether it was true women my age in Poland were considered too old to marry, and their other friend who had once brought me a packet of sweets to the centre. One afternoon, on my way back to my hostel, I saw those three entering a pub together. They all looked clean and fresh and lovely after their visit to the Day Centre. They noticed me too and suggested I come along with them. I refused, mostly because having paid for a couple more weeks at my hostel I did not even have enough money for a drink. Indeed, after my hostel breakfast, a leftover sandwich from the day centre at the end of my shift was my only meal those days. I often felt hungry. As I watched the men walk into the pub I could not afford, it dawned on me that among the poor of London, I was not much richer.

***

One afternoon, somebody waved to me from across the street in Kingsland Road, North-east London, "Hello! How are you?"

I recognised the man from the hotel reception who had taken my Polish phone number.

"Oh, hello," I smiled broadly. I was happy to see a familiar face in this new country full of strangers.

He scampered across the road between some cars.

"Did I tell you my name?" he grinned, "My name is Kenny. Where are you coming from? Have you found a job?"

"No, I have not. I am volunteering at a day centre."

"And I am on my way from the bank here. I had to deposit some cash for the hotel. It is a responsible job to deal with money, you know. I do a lot of things for the hotel. They trust me."

"Looks like they do."

"Do you always walk alone? You should be very careful on your own. There are a lot of dangerous people here."

"I am not afraid of dangerous people. Dangerous people are good to me." I smiled.

"Are they?" Kenny perused me for a while. "Look, if you still need a job in three weeks from now, we should have a vacancy for you," he said, "One boy is leaving the hotel. The boy is from Cyprus, and I am from Cyprus too, so he told me his plans, but he asked me not to tell anyone else. Therefore, don't tell anyone. Just come to the hotel in three weeks from now."

***

It was Arslan, a Turkish engineer based in South London, who tipped me off in the summer of 2003 that a Mediterranean and Middle Eastern deli in the Croydon area was looking for staff. I had met Arslan online, through the ICQ messenger, while in Poland. He was a wonderful person, very peaceful and entirely focused on his religion, Islam. Perhaps this was a reason why we never became close friends, since I was not keen to discuss converting, and I always felt uneasy during our conversations, which perpetually revolved around God and religion. I liked Arslan as a person though and I trusted him, so I contacted him after arriving in London.

Arslan went to Croydon, to the deli, with me. He had me wait a few steps away in the shop owner's view as he spoke to them about me. That was my whole recruitment process for the vacancy, with Arslan speaking for me. He got me my first paying UK job. The shop was to pay me £150.00 per week. Arslan also lent me his own money for my start here. I think I borrowed as much as £400 for my home deposit from him, and I made sure I gave every penny back to him as soon as I could.

I moved to the Croydon area. Somebody had told me South London was different from North London. One was richer and one had more immigrants. I tried to spot some differences as I moved, but the London I knew never looked any richer anywhere. I did not see any high-end retail outlets, probably not because there weren't any around, but because I automatically ignored them as being far beyond my reach. What I did see was the shutters of small food shops with delivery crates to unload, or some litter in the streets that needed tidying up.

Riding on a bus through Streatham, I noticed an old graveyard with its stones partially covered with moss. I spontaneously got off my bus. One more passenger hopped off just after me before the bus moved on. I walked between the graves, crouching down beside the stones to read the old inscriptions. There was the kind of peace you find in a deep forest, combined with the loneliness of a big city street. Suddenly, I saw the man from my bus, standing nearby and staring at me. I quickly made my way towards the pavement.

"I didn't want to scare you," he said to me, "I'm sorry. Are you Polish?"

"How on earth do you know?" I asked.

He moved his hand in front of his eyes.

"Something about the upper part of your face."

I later learnt my almond shaped eyes were different from rounder west-European eyes. Londoners are often good at guessing your ethnicity. I am still learning the skill. The man had a tanned complexion with dark eyes and black hair. As we walked away from the graveyard back into the busy street, I felt safer and more comfortable, and I listened attentively. He was from France, where his parents had migrated from Morocco, although he did not know Morocco and called himself French.

"Why don't we sit down here for a while?" he suggested as we were passing a coffee shop.

The tables outside the coffee shop looked inviting. We

sat down at one of those little tables and had a cup of coffee or hot chocolate together. I also ordered myself a croissant.

"It is a French word, isn't it? How do you pronounce it? "/Krosau/"? I asked, trying to sound French and remember the silent "t" at the end.

"In Paris we say, "/kruasou/", but then of course there are so many different accents," said the man, clearly not wanting to sound critical of my linguistic efforts. What diplomatic flair he had! We said good-bye soon after that, but it was nice to have met.

CHAPTER THREE – THE INTERNAUT

The Clinical Psychologist placed a box of tissues near me; it was 2007 and we were in central London. I was not crying, but tissues were routinely provided to patients for their appointments. There was no special couch in the room like in the clichéd version a psychotherapy patient would recline on. There were standard chairs, however the chairs had a soft seat and a soft back rest in cheerful pastel colours. All the colour schemes in modern therapy rooms are designed to lift the patient's spirits. If there are curtains at the window, there will be some cheery colours in the curtain print. The artwork will show either the nature in bloom or abstract compositions of blue, red, or other bright colours. There will be no grey or broken brownish colour schemes.

"I too have been through psychosis," the Clinical Psychologist said to me. Then she may have felt insecure about her own confession because she quickly added, "Of course, I was not ill for as long as you were. I was only psychotic for one day."

Her words, "of course not for as long as you," felt a little uncomfortable to me, however meeting a post-psychotic professional was still a powerfully validating experience for the timid new post-psychotic patient that I was. I contemplated how collected and focused she was, and despite the fact she put lots of effort in my consultation, nothing she later said could match the uplifting impact her own story had on me.

I had met a number of different mental health professionals

by now. One mentioned her upcoming holiday to me, and it felt like she must have been thinking mainly about this holiday during my appointment, because there were factual errors in the summary of my consultation that I later received in writing from her.

Not this Clinical Psychologist though. This one listened attentively, taking accurate notes, and I appreciated being listened to. Of course, she asked about my childhood. I talked about my childhood home, about my school, about my parents. When I read her summary later, I discovered that my family had been described as "emotionally undemonstrative." Those words struck me. I had never thought about us that way, but she had a point. The family just got on with things without expressing a lot of feelings.

***

They often say people develop mental health problems after a challenging childhood. That would not be the case for me. My parents were caring. My childhood was happy and relatively carefree. Of course, I lived in an Orwellian-style dystopia, but so did everyone around me in communist Poland at the time.

Although I did my schooling in the eighties, I did still experience communism to a degree. In 1980 my parents asked us not to mention at school that we had a typewriter at home. My understanding as a child was that the Militia did not like people with typewriters. Those people often typed anti-government leaflets through carbonated paper for multiple copies. Mum explained to us they might accuse us of something we had not done.

It was only many years later that I read some paperwork prepared by Dad for his workplace. Dad had been the chairman of the 1970 Strike Committee in his power plant in southern Poland, and his written instructions were to organise their power cuts in a well-co-ordinated way that would ensure uninterrupted power supplies to the nearby hospitals for the medical equipment. Mum kept this paperwork. Dad had escaped the Militia during the 1980 arrests, but he had later been regularly called in for interrogations at a Militia station where he had been beaten. He had been offered asylum in Canada, but he stayed in Poland. I will never understand why Dad never joined his friends abroad. Instead, he had withdrawn from politics, and we moved to another town, to mum's old family house. Dad was only awarded a knight's cross posthumously.

***

The fall of communism in Poland shaped my early professional life as I became an English language teacher rather young. Russian language was no longer the main foreign language to teach in Polish schools. The English language shot to popularity, but there was a shortage of fully trained English language teachers. That was how they offered me my first official school teaching job in 1994 when I was 21.

Teaching to teenagers, I was often amazed at how much wisdom they already had.

I once tried to get my pupils to talk about some dating agency clients described in their English course books. "Do you think she will find her dream date?"

"No. Not really."

"Why not?"

"Because you have to keep an open mind when meeting new people and she doesn't. She has already decided what the man should look like, and what his job should be; she has planned everything about him and now she is trying to find somebody who will fill those shoes. She will not find that man. You have to allow the other person to be themselves, to be unique."

I started working with the school's oldest group of 19-year-old boys when I was 23.

"Was that a pupil of yours?" asked me one female friend from my school days after a young man greeted me in the street, "You must be kidding me, do you have pupils like that? So dishy!"

Things like receiving porn stories from pupils instead of decent homework and all the other difficult behaviours that can be aimed at a young teacher came later in my working life. My oldest boys, in fact, were genuinely kind to me. An anonymous bunch of roses was delivered to my family home on Teachers Day. It was common for Polish adults to live with their parents, and I also lived in my family home in my 20s. One evening, several 19-year-old boys turned up on my doorstep wearing smart suits and holding a spare theatre ticket for me. My father opened the door to them. I was out at the time, fortunately, so I was spared the heartbreak of having to personally decline a night out together. In a way, they were a challenge, too though. My biggest challenge with them was to never fall in love. They may have been adults already, but they were still at school, and I would have been sacked for getting too close to any of them.

My oldest group of pupils graduated in 1997, and a few persuaded me to create my first email address so we could keep in touch after they left for university. Before I first got online, I had to buy a modem for my new computer. I dismantled the cover of my personal computer and attached my new modem with screws to the structure inside. Then the computer would not turn on, so I finally phoned a hardware service centre. The engineer arrived at my place and plugged my computer back into the electric socket under my desk. It worked. Then he gave me a bill for his attendance.

The dial-up Internet connection was expensive in Poland in 1997, and I spent a large chunk of my salary on it. The connection was charged per minute, like a phone call. The Internet was new, and it seemed to be full of international people seeking contacts abroad.

"I am from Balkaria", somebody wrote to me in English via ICQ messenger.

"Did you mean Bulgaria?" I replied.

"Oh no, don't do that to me," he said, "you are only in

Poland, but you are behaving as if you were somewhere in America! I am here in Balkaria, in the Caucasus!"

"Ah the Caucasus! Yes, of course, I know where you are," I replied.

He sent me his photo. Dark smiling eyes, dark hair under a thick warm fur hood, and heavy snow weighing down a branch over his head and spreading everywhere in sight are the Balkaria I know.

***

Eddie was a good runner. That strength had spared him jail in his teenage years. Born black in 1977 in apartheid-torn South Africa, he had actively participated in the early 1990s demonstrations. After one protest, young Eddie had managed to run halfway to another town by the time the local police came searching for him at his home and neighbourhood.

I loved Eddie's story. My dad had been chased and bothered by the Polish Militia in communist times, so I felt very strongly about people who had the courage to peacefully oppose oppressive regimes. I thought there were some parallels between our families. Eddie and I had both experienced the fall of our respective countries' regimes during our teenage years. Eddie was 17 when they formed the democratic South African government in 1994. I was 16 when communism collapsed in Poland in 1989. People had been killed during both regimes. Eddie and I both were given opportunities our parents had not had. The two of us met online in the noughties when the world had become a digitally connected global village. I admired Eddie's drive to chase his dreams and how he had managed to leave behind his life of poverty through his brains, ambition, and focus that had landed him a corporate job. He was always reading books, and I felt as if I had always known him. There seemed to be some deep familiarity about him, and we both resolved to learn as much as we could about each other and about our backgrounds.

***

Eddie had various stories to tell. For instance, he told me that, during apartheid, black South Africans had been allowed to do certain university courses – although they had not been allowed to study the law, medicine, or engineering. Those faculties had been the exclusive, potentially empowering three.

Eddie's given names were Nkosiyabo Eduard, an African name followed by an Afrikaner name, but he used an English nickname instead. His black South African colleagues also only spoke English at work, in the early noughties, despite everyone being able to speak Afrikaans. Both English and Afrikaans were officially in use, as were nine African languages: Sepedi, Sesotho, Setswana, siSwati, Tshivenda, Xitsonga, isiNdebele, isiXhosa, and isiZulu. So, there are eleven official languages in the so-called Rainbow Nation.

My favourite story, however, was about their Women's Day. Women's Day in South Africa is not in March as it is in so many other countries. In SA, it is on 9th August. When you look online nowadays, you may read that this is "for the memory of 20,000 women's march to the government buildings in 1956." Eddie, however, told it differently to me. He said there had been lots of earlier marches by men who had been shot at. The authorities had been ruthless, and a lot of men had died. Therefore, out of despair, women had organised their own march. When the governor had learnt about women marching, rather than having them shot at, he had left the government building through the back door. (Actually, it may have been the Prime Minister rather than the Governor-General. I may have confused the title). In either way, the oppressor leaving through his back door was the punchline of the story, the way they remembered it there. "The power of women," Eddie commented.

I enjoyed reading Eddie's emails. They were informative, if not intellectual, and it was fascinating to me to see his different perspective of the world, which was like a fresh breeze.

***

The feeling I should protect the younger people from myself was ingrained in me by the time I met Eddie. I told him that regardless of the physical distance between our countries, I could never be his girlfriend, because he was too young. Eddie was four years younger than I. We may have both been in our 20s, but he was the age of my "little" beloved former pupils.

"I honestly cannot believe that I am getting turned down, just because I was born too late!" he exclaimed. "You know I cannot help when I was born."

I laughed, and I could not help liking him more and more.

*****

Many years later, right after my first psychotic episode, a Polish psychologist had me take a multiple-choice test.

"Your test results show you have a schizoaffective personality", she said.

"What does that mean? Has my psychosis altered my personality?

"No, this is just how you are. You have always been this way."

I thought for a while.

"But if I always had a personality disorder, didn't I do remarkably well until my thirties?"

She did not reply.

I am of course not an expert to judge whether my personality is standard or not. But I do believe certain events in my life may have amplified the force of my breakdown, and some of my habits may have caused it. Perhaps my lonely long-distance marriage contributed to my breakdown, and my experience of harassment and bullying may have added to it. I also may have relied too much on myself though, instead of looking for help. I used to feel I could take on the world of challenges, although some of those challenges proved too much for me. As I share my story, you can see where things went wrong.

CHAPTER FOUR – THE GOOD WOMAN

The World Food Deli in South London sold a vast variety of products in 2003. "The butcher, the baker, the candlestick maker" works as a description of what the shop was like. We may not have sold candlesticks as such, but apart from bread and meat we did stock water pipes, warm blankets, tableware, and shimmery pictures of the Al Kaaba stone and mosque.

I had come to the UK with strong plans to refine my English and be a better teacher and translator back in Poland. However, I sometimes only spoke my broken Turkish at the World Food Deli. My colleagues laughed, saying I was going to master my Turkish instead. I had previously done some Turkish language studies at Cracow's Jagiellonian University in Poland, and I had just enough knowledge to understand some insults, for instance.

"Kadın'dan nefret ediyorum", meaning "I hate this woman", was one comment about me by one of the shop owners after I insisted on an urgent delivery of packaging for some cakes I was selling.

"Zeytinler ne pis," meaning "How rubbish these olives are," commented some teenage customers on the produce I was selling.

At first, I worked at the bakery and confectionery counter. The white baguettes covered with a thick layer of sesame seeds were called çörek by Turks and somoon by Greeks; the two ethnic groups each considered these baguettes their own. The long, thin Iranian barbari bread had to be folded in half or it would not fit into any bag we had. I kept on learning, and I loved it.

"Where do you say these come from?", asked one customer about our Mediterranean doughnuts. "Do you say they are Greek, or do you say they are Turkish?"

"They are so popular in the whole region it is really hard to tell nowadays where exactly they originated from," I bluffed, trying to be diplomatic, although I did not know.

"Some olives can be a bit old here," a lovely Turkish girl, Nurgül, confided while she was training me during my first days at work. "You will learn to recognise those that are less fresh. Naturally, we cannot tell the customers that some of our olives are old, so what I normally say is. 'These olives have a rather strong taste; therefore, you may want to try some before you buy them.' Then the decision is theirs, but people usually listen to what I tell them."

After Nurgül had left the shop, I soon learned which olive boxes on my display to warn against. They were the ones I had had to wash the mould off upon first opening the large cans. I used Nurgül's exact words about those olives.

"These olives have a rather strong taste; therefore, you may want to try some before you buy them," I said.

People who were as new to olive tasting as I was, usually went for other produce. However, some Mediterranean and Middle Eastern people were angry with me.

"Are you suggesting I do not know my olives?" some of them said, "I have been eating olives every day since I was a child. You are not here to try and sell me things of your own choice, but to give me what I choose. See, give me one of those olives. Umm, they are excellent. They are exactly how I remember them from my childhood."

"Did you know that the chickens they sell here are not halal?" asked a customer with a long dark beard, wearing a white robe.

"I can ask my manager to talk to you if you would like to speak about our chickens," I said.

"No, don't do that," he protested, "Don't call anyone.

They would lie to me, and I do not want them to lie. See this vein in your chicken that I have just bought. There is some blood in this vein, and this is how I know they had broken this chicken's neck. Had they killed it in the halal way, there would be no blood left. I just thought I would tell you because, of all the staff here, you are one that may have not known."

Near my counters, people even asked me repeatedly if the cheese that I had cut was halal, even though I could not think of any kind of cheese in the world that would not be halal.

Some Turkish women were sceptical of my looks: "Yabancıya konuşmam" ("I will not speak to the foreigner"), they muttered. I just smiled at them in silence.

I said to my manager Emir that my pale looks might be driving some customers away from my counter, but he just laughed.

***

I had needed a room quickly then, in the summer of 2003, for my new job in Croydon, and I had circled two local single room ads in my copy of Loot newspaper. One of the ads was for a room in a two-bedroom flat to share with two gay men on condition you were "gay-friendly". I was quite eager to phone those two as I thought living together with them could be fun and surely no-one in there would pester me for sex. I wished I had applied to share home with those two men. However, I pondered this expression they had used, "gay-friendly". Since I am not a natural English speaker, I simply did not understand this phrase. I thought you might need to be gay to live there. The other ad, "room in a family house", was written in plain language that I recognised from my old handbooks, and I understood every word. I chose the family house ad. That was how I moved into this Pakistani family's Thornton Heath house. The father of the family told me to keep all my future cooking utensils inside my bedroom; he had lined the shelves in my room with newspapers in advance. There was a bed, a table, and one wooden hard chair. I was unable to sit on my wooden chair for too long after a day's physical lifting and prolonged standing at work, or my back hurt. Their plush living room was for the family use only.

I still had no radio nor TV nor a computer in the UK, and my mobile phone was a basic handset with no internet facility, so I had no access to any entertainment in my room. I would lie on my bed in silence until I fell asleep. I only lasted two weeks in that room.

"You are not going anywhere," my landlord said to me.

"Yes, I am," I said, but I left my tiny deposit with him when I moved out.

I moved straight to my new Turkish manager's home, a two-bedroom house that I got to share with a few Turkish friends. As my deposit, I gave them the £400 I had got off Arslan.

There were two men sleeping on the two sofas in the living room downstairs. My manager Emir was one of them, and his best friend Eren, also Turkish, was the other. Eren was temporarily unemployed, and he sometimes cooked dinner for our whole household before the rest of us got back from work. I loved the British TV in their living room, which we all spent our evenings in. I loved their comfy sofas I could rest my weary spine against while having a chat or watching TV. Upstairs, there were bedrooms for girls only. One girl was my colleague Nuray, who had come to London for a short time to practice her English before building her established career back in Turkey. I shared one of the two upstairs bedrooms with Nuray. The other bedroom was occupied by another Turkish girl, Nehir, who was not working with us, but who was Eren's cousin. Nehir was dating an English boy who had joined the British Army. She was planning to marry her soldier, and she often stayed at her boyfriend's mother's house rather than with us. I felt happy around my colleagues in their house. They said I should feel free to use whatever food there was in the fridge, and, as I bought my own food,

I also made sure to never buy anything containing pork or gelatine or alcohol, so all my food would be suitable for them, too. We shared it all.

Nuray, Emir and I worked for the same shop, however we usually travelled to work at different times. One morning Emir was late, and he drove me to work with him. Our colleagues were gathered outside the shutters at the front of the deli.

"Good morning, Mister Emir," they greeted our manager.

"Good morning," Emir replied.

"Good morning," I smiled toward our colleagues, but they did not reply to me.

The boys looked down in silence when I looked at them. All my Middle Eastern male colleagues stopped talking to me after that morning when they had seen me in Emir's car. I started feeling uneasy at my workplace and I did not know how to handle my irrational but ongoing feeling of rejection.

One male colleague, Ali, finally asked me directly in the storeroom downstairs: "Tell me, do you sleep with him?" He was helping me pick up some large cans of food.

I was relieved to be asked. That way, I got my chance to deny it. I explained to Ali that I shared my room with Nuray, the Muslim checkout girl everyone respected, and that we both rented our room from Emir. My male colleagues soon started speaking to me again.

***

I remembered Kenny and his words about an upcoming vacancy at the hotel. Three weeks had passed. I was no longer searching for a job, but I decided to go and say thank you anyhow.

There was a middle-aged man sitting at the hotel reception desk.

"Excuse me, is Kenny around?" I asked.

"He is not," said a man in a way that I felt was abrupt, "Did you have an appointment with him? What is it regarding?"

"No, I did not, I'm sorry, it's nothing important," I said.

"Don't go," said the man, "I would like to talk to you."

The man brought me a chair over and asked me to sit down. I did.

"Kenny has left," he said. "He has stolen a lot of money from the hotel and disappeared. The police are looking for him. If you know where he could be, you need to tell us or the police. Do you know where he could have gone?"

"I don't know," I said quietly with my eyes wide open. I was shocked and I felt for this man who was leaning against the reception desk.

"Did he leave you? Were you in a relationship with him?" the hotel manager or owner asked me more softly.

"No, I wasn't," I replied. I told my story to the man.

"So, he told you there was somebody leaving our hotel?"

"Yes, he did. Was that true?"

"No, it wasn't." The man paused, "Are you still looking for a job?"

"No, I'm not. I already have a job. I just came here on my day off to say thank you."

I later thought about it, and I realised that indeed there had been "a boy from Cyprus" leaving the hotel. It had been Kenny. Kenny may have planned for himself to be replaced by me.

***

I refrained from food and drink during the month of Ramadan in late 2003 as I was around various colleagues who fasted. On the first day I forgot, and I tried some of the salad I was making. Later I simply stayed focused and managed to remember not to put anything in my mouth for the rest of the day.

"What religion are you?" some colleagues asked me, "Are you fasting?"

"I am Christian," I said, "But I am keeping you company."

It may have been one of the easier Ramadans in Europe,

because it was winter, and the days were short. We were still at work when the daily fasting time ended. They said you traditionally break your Ramadan fasting with water and dates. If I was alone in my section, one of the butcher boys would come over to my area in the evenings with an open box of dates, to let me know it was the correct time to break the fasting. They also placed some open boxes of free dates for the customers at the entrance to the shop to celebrate those moments.

After daytimes of fasting, my body wanted to make up for the shortage of food. During Ramadan 2003 I sometimes ate a loaf of bread a night, after work. Our deli sales went up. We had to introduce limits in our bakery section, as a lot of our fasting customers had large meals in the evenings, with lots of guests. I was not allowed to sell more than ten loaves of bread per customer, and the limitation was genuine since some customers requested more, especially of the large flat oval Turkish "pide" bread.

***

One day a female colleague said to me at our Deli, "Aidan from the vegetable section asked me to speak to you for him. He would rather speak to your family, but you do not have a family here, so he asked me instead, because we work together, and because I am your friend. He thinks you are a good woman, and he would like you to be with him."

"What do you mean, 'be with him'?" I asked.

"Well, to be with him," she repeated, looking at me steadily with her big eyes.

"Well, I don't even know him... I have never spoken to him..."

"That's what I thought. I told him you would say no because you are a good woman. But I finally agreed to speak to you because you really have no family here. That's men, you see. I can't believe them. They are fasting through the day, but they keep all that shit in their heads at the same time!"

I never got together with Aidan, but I did later talk to him a lot. I enjoyed listening to his stories of Iraq. He showed me his scars from the bullets, as he had spent most of his time fighting in the mountains.

One day I dragged Aidan out to a pub near our workplace. Because his religion did not permit drinking alcohol, we ordered some fruit juice and sat at a small table on tall chairs. It was nice chatting together. At some point Aidan looked round, saying,

"This moment. It would have never happened in Iraq. We would not be allowed to do this."

I thought for a while, then looked at our glasses, which were half-full of juice.

"Except we are not doing anything," I answered.

"Ah you don't understand," he waved his hand, "Iraq is completely different. Even I would not be able to go out to a pub after work, not to mention a woman. In Iraq, if people saw a woman on her own, everyone would think she had got lost."

Aidan invited me to dinner with his cousins at their home. We squatted down on their carpet, and they served some delicious food on a tablecloth that was spread between us on the carpeted floor. The house was filled with the scent of rose petals from an air freshener plugged in an electric socket. When Aidan left us for a while, his brother stood up and showed me a photo of a dark-eyed woman wearing a hijab.

"Do you know who this is?" he asked.

"This must be Aidan's wife," I answered, and because the brother looked distressed to me, I added, "She is very pretty."

The woman in the photo truly was good-looking. Aidan's brother went silent, and he sat down. Aidan had told me he was married. His wife lived in Iraq and apparently, she had insisted she did not want to join Aidan "in the land of Satan", which was what she thought the United Kingdom was. Aidan had told me they were getting divorced, although clearly his family saw things differently.

***

One of my colleagues was Yargül, a young Kurdish woman from Turkey. Just like Ali in the storeroom, Yargül also asked me if I was sleeping with Emir, but she did it in a more delicate way.

"Do you sleep in the same room as Mister Emir?" were her words.

I did not find her question offensive, as I knew Yargül was curious about life outside her home or the shop. I explained I slept in the same room as Nuray.

"Did you drink alcohol when you met the colleagues outside work last week?" Yargül asked on another day, "Did the Turkish girls do that, too?"

"I do sometimes drink alcohol, but last week we didn't. We sat down at the tables outside a coffee shop, and we had some coffee together," I said.

"I wish I could meet for a coffee like this," she said, "but my father wouldn't let me."

Another time, as she spoke about a seaside, she said,

"My brother could even bathe in the sea. I could not. I wish I could bathe in the sea."

Yargül told me she was planning to go away with her family. After she stopped coming to work, one man asked me about her as I was serving at the bakery section.

"I am Yargül's father," he said, "She has run away with her mother and sister. Do you know where she is?"

Even if I knew where Yargül was, I would not have told him. I silently wished the girls best of luck with their move, and I was proud of Yargül. Her father, in turn, told me he had a British passport and was happy to remarry. He asked if I had a boyfriend.

"Oh, I am not looking for a husband," I giggled, trying to say no in a polite way.

"And you should," he said.

Then I had to fetch some crates of more fresh bread from downstairs, and Yargül's father disappeared from my counter.

***

Eddie, who I had met online while in Poland, came from South Africa to London to visit me on tourist visa. We had been exchanging regular emails for months, praising each other, and swearing about how deeply we felt for each other. Eddie had thus become my long-distance boyfriend, and, as I came out to meet him at Heathrow airport for the first time, I felt I ought to like him in person.

Fortunately, he looked good. Tall and slim, with a sincere broad smile, he captured my heart very quickly.

One night as Eddie was staying in a Croydon hotel, he walked me to my South London home. He just missed his last bus to his hotel that night. Not wanting to spend any money on cabs, he ran along the street until he caught up with his bus. As he boarded the bus at the next stop, some passengers clapped their hands, and the driver told him cheerfully to "just keep on running".

CHAPTER FIVE – THE NOMAD

My spirit was not yet beaten in 2004. I did not yet foresee the weakness that was going to creep onto my life in the years to come. In January 2004, my UK student visa expired, and I went back to Poland. I found a technical school with a maternity cover available till June. I taught English to groups of teenage boys again. There was a group of 18-year-old boys, one of whom told me on behalf of their group they would not learn English, because they could not, and that I should "accept" the fact they were "stupid" and back off.

"Yes, you can. And I am going to prove to you that you can," was my reply.

I asked them to do an exercise for me one day in class, to use various English modal verbs, which are words like "must, should, needn't, mustn't". I got them to describe their ideal partners with those modal verbs. First of all, I let it be their choice. Had I directly asked them to talk about their dream partners, they would have refused to, I knew this, so I gave them a range of topics to choose from. I remember that describing a good teacher, or another working person of their choice, were on that list of possible topics for them to select, but of course everybody chose to describe their ideal girlfriend instead. I asked them to write down their ideas. To make things easier for them, everyone was to write down just five sentences, with five different modal verbs.

"I would like to read my composition aloud," said one boy from the back row of tables.

I asked him to go on.

"My ideal girlfriend," he read, "must have big breasts."

A lot of other boys roared with laughter. I stood there silently, with my hands rolled in tight fists in my pockets. "It is your own fault, woman," I thought to myself, "encouraging them to talk about girlfriends." I did not know what to say. The boys were still giggling, and I became intensely aware of the fact that I was the only woman in the classroom, and my own chest was perhaps more modest than one he had started describing. I found the whole situation embarrassing. Then again, I thought, I was there to teach them English and not to be thinking about whatever shape my own body was.

"Go on," I said, digging my nails into my hands in my pockets and preparing for another blow.

The boys stared silently at me and then at him again.

"Actually, that is my whole composition," he said, "I have already finished reading."

The other boys burst out laughing again.

"I asked you to write five sentences", I said. "What you have written is grammatically correct. Go on."

Another cheeky boy was waving his hands toward me, also from the back row. "I want to read mine. Let me read mine."

"Oh no, not him", I thought to myself, "this one is going to describe what she should look like below her waist". I was already regretting giving them a topic like that to write on. There was no sensible way of escaping though, so I told him to go on, too.

"She shouldn't take drugs," he read aloud, "She must love me..."

When he read all his five sentences, which were so lovely and charming, and fortunately also correct, so I did not have to correct anything, I grabbed their register and put down a very good grade against his name, for his participation in class and for that exercise.

Nearly everyone read aloud their five sentences, and they were fantastic, and a lot of the boys got their very good grades on the day.

"She needn't be beautiful," one boy wrote. That was immensely sweet to hear.

"She mustn't betray me," said another boy, and I asked how he meant it, whether he meant sleeping with someone else or if he meant something different.

He said he meant sleeping with someone else.

"They have this separate expression in English then", I said, "to cheat on someone". The boys asked me to write that down on the blackboard and they too wrote it down in their notebooks, "She mustn't cheat on me."

The lesson seemed to be turning for the better; I was finding my way through to them. Then the first boy got back to me.

"Do you really think I meant what I said?" he asked, "How could you possibly think that was for real?"

He was angry with me. But I was already feeling tired, enough emotions for me in that class, and I did not want to analyse things with him. He was 18 years old anyway, not 8, and my understanding was that he had deliberately tried to sabotage my lesson in the first place.

"I only know as much about you as you tell me," I said in my dry voice, and the subject was closed.

He never forgave me, that first boy, ever at all.

***

Poland joined the EU in June 2004, and I could come back without a visa to London where I had left my heart. I returned to World Food Deli, where I stayed until my brother Radek visited me in London. Radek is four years younger than me. We shared a lot of secrets in our childhood, such as one of a five-year-old Radek pulling me away from a pond after my shoes got stuck in the mud, with a bunch of rushes he had picked up to use like a rope. In London, Radek persuaded me to look for a new job, one with proper tax and holidays paid.

"What are you even doing at this place?" he asked.

The World Food Deli paid me £150 a week, which was

enough for me to survive on, as I only paid £50 a week for my bed in shared room, but the shop owners had me working six 12-hour shifts a week for that money. The hourly minimum wage was £4.20 in 2003, rising to £4.50 in October 2003 through most of 2004, but I did not earn even half of that. I earned £2.08 per hour at the Deli. No tax and no national insurance were paid for me. I never reported it anywhere. I did not even know how to report it.

Many years later, I came across a Polish community shop in North London that also offered to pay me below the minimum wage. I think some of those stores use the fact they speak minority languages to function as separate states within the official state. They hire workers who often have no English, and they create a dysfunctional sub-universe for their workers.

Radek and I went together to Ravenscourt Park, west London, on my day off to look at various job ads displayed behind the window of a Polish shop. It was a famous spot among London's Polish community at the time, and Radek had read about it back in Poland. The glass wall of this specific shop indeed was full of little papers with different ads printed or hand-written on them. Lots of low-paying jobs were advertised there. I liked an ad seeking a mature lady to run a launderette. I phoned Wasif the boss from my pay-as-you-go British mobile number.

"Hello, I'm calling to apply for the job at a launderette," I said.

"And how old are you?" Wasif asked.

"I am 31."

"That's good. When can you come to our head office for an interview?"

The following week, I went to Park Royal, North-west London, to meet Wasif for an interview. The company owned a chain of launderettes; their head office was above a dry-cleaning and commercial laundry processing floor. They wanted to learn more about my level of English. They gave me the task of typing a letter to an imaginary customer in relation to my deli job. I drafted a letter praising my deli's range of patisserie products available for parties. I invited this imaginary customer to visit us at my cakes section to try different kinds of baklava and other traditional Mediterranean and Middle Eastern cookies, and I also included some practical information in that letter, about the deposit required for baking trays that was refundable upon return of the empty clean trays. Wasif loved the letter, especially the fragment praising traditional Middle Eastern cookies, and he read aloud this fragment to his wife, Kaitlin. That was how I learnt Wasif's family were originally from Iran. Kaitlin also liked the letter and, rather than the launderette job, I was offered a telephone-based customer service job in their head office.

***

My interview at Five Stars the laundry was in the late morning of a bright sunny day. I walked back from it feeling victorious. I had been offered a real minimum wage job. I was elated at the thought of a new opportunity opening its door to me. I felt I could fly, and I spread my arms wide while enjoying the moment. Suddenly a man appeared at the side of the pavement, and he grabbed my handbag, trying to tug it off my stretched arm. I had my passport and all my wages in my bag. I knew that without my passport I would not be able to travel to South Africa to Eddie's, which I was planning to do, so I fought for my bag. In fact, I simply held tight on to my handbag's strap.

The mugger spun with my bag in his hands and, still holding the long strap, I swirled around him like a puppet. The man then punched me on the side of my head, cracking my ear slightly, but my hands stayed clenched against the strap. I could see only one other pedestrian in the street. He was headed in the opposite direction, wearing his large earphones. I screamed for help, but he could not hear me. Then, I was saved by two unlikely heroes. One elderly grey-haired lady and one gentleman who had difficulty walking both stopped their cars and started walking toward us. Some other motorists were also forced to stop behind them. My attacker ran away, having thrown my handbag down on the ground beside me, with my hands still clenching its long leather strap.

"Are you alright?" my two heroes asked me in clear native English. "Would you like a lift?"

I was shaken, so I did want a lift, and the lady dropped me off at the nearest underground station, at North Acton. I never forgot those two people and their enormous courage and selflessness.

The laundry gave me some homework. I had to learn how to use Excel spreadsheets before the start of my job. I had one month for my self-study. I quit World Food Deli and spent the following month in South Africa with Eddie, who downloaded some Excel tutorials for me to go through on my own at his home while he was at work.

The World Food Deli was one of my very few former workplaces where none of my former colleagues kept in touch with me. As if everyone wanted to forget it.

***

From my childhood, I thought one day I would want to find a man to have and raise my children with: the traditional way of life.

"So, have you chosen your boyfriend yet?" asked some visiting family members in my late teens. They were clearly hoping for the family to multiply in all directions through all offspring.

I didn't have a boyfriend until my 20s, though. The truth is, I wanted some special, unusual, out-of-this-world kind of love. The boys I knew were not out of this world and I was naïve to think that one day I would meet someone I would fall head over heels in love with, in a thrilling way, leading a lifetime of fireworks.

"Kasia has always been picky," my sister's husband said

to my mum about me once. "Some of my mates wanted to go out with her, but she always turned everyone down."

In my 20s I eventually started dating, although I pulled out quickly each time.

"What is it you want, Kasia?" asked one young man I had started dating, "Surely, we can try to make things work for us, for you."

"No, I'm sorry, I can't," I said. "This is just not it."

"Not what? How do you mean not it?"

"I don't know, it is simply not it."

I couldn't describe what I meant. I just vaguely felt that, after all, it wasn't the exciting big love I had dreamt about.

When I met Eddie online, our long-distance conversations were all we had. Those were stimulating, clever, sincere talks for me. We had never faced the little mundane challenges life brings together. We had never had to accept and forgive each other's imperfections. I probably fooled myself into believing that life with Eddie would be free from the prosaic components and only built on the excitement of our inspired interactions. There was no room for any disappointments or disagreements in our online relationship across different hemispheres.

If my vision of Eddie lacked some deeper knowledge of his character, I substituted those elements with my dreams and hopes of how he was. I felt I had finally found the big love I had so far only read about. I now struggle to believe it myself, but that is how I was.

CHAPTER SIX – THE FOREIGNER

My dad was no longer alive when I got engaged to Eddie, but my mum was openly worried about my choice.

"You hardly know him," she said.

She also was concerned there could be some cultural differences between me and the foreign man I was planning to marry so quickly. My mother had never been abroad, but she was an avid reader, and she was discouraged by some of what she had read in Poland about distant countries. When Eddie visited us in Poland, one afternoon as we were talking, my mum askcd Eddie if people in his country believed in magic. I froze. Eddie was a university-trained professional, and I felt my mum's question on magic was offensive. However, astoundingly he said yes, a lot of the people certainly did.

"Not me," he said, "and not my father either, but lots of people do and my father jokes a lot about that. Now it seems to be fading in a way as the electricity is advancing for instance, among other things. The magic men hate the electricity. They say it interferes with their magic and that it diminishes their powers. But they are still there. My father always says he likes his electricity very much. My family are on the electricity's side."

My mum later returned Eddie's honesty.

"Polish people also used to dream of colonising Africa, we were not better than that," she said., "In the 18th century, they wanted to establish a Polish colony in Madagascar."

"Why Madagascar?" asked Eddie, "There is nothing there. There are no resources."

"Are there not?" My mum laughed and added that Eddie was exceptionally intelligent.

Mum, my brother and I worried Eddie might encounter some unpleasant behaviours while in Poland. We did not know anyone black in Poland, but we had heard stories of some black men getting beaten in Polish streets from the media. Just in case, the three of us agreed my brother should always be near Eddie in the streets. Wherever Eddie and I went, we were as if "casually" accompanied by my brother. To our relief, apart from some people staring, nothing bad happened. On the contrary, when Eddie and I went to church together, the people standing near us all wanted to shake hands with Eddie, some of them forgetting to shake hands with me, as he was the star, not me.

***

Later in South Africa we drew even more attention. A group of black men shouted "Mrs Zimbabwe" at me in the street for being a poor white without a car.

I stayed in South Africa with Eddie for a few weeks. If I were to compare South Africa to anywhere else that I had been to, it would be to Arizona, U.S.A, which I had briefly visited before. The sky was as intensely blue, and the sun was as big and strong. I sometimes felt dizzy from the sun. The earth in South Africa was a rusty colour, different from our Polish black earth, and I kept that rusty reddish dust on my shoes with sentiment and pride after returning to London.

Eddie talked to me about all the things we could see, trying to explain his country to me.

"There are mines in this area," he said as we drove past some rocks. "Lots of these resources are still owned by the British. The lorries that enter gold or diamond mines are weighed on very delicate scales, so that no amount of the precious resources can be smuggled out."

We passed some people near small huts with corrugated steel for roofs.

"It is extremely hot in those huts," Eddie continued, "but they are temporary homes only. Those workers have their shacks in other towns."

Eddie's parents lived in a township shack. Townships had been built spontaneously, and of course illegally, around towns and cities during the apartheid regime by the black people who had nowhere else to live. After the fall of apartheid, the land was divided and the tiny lots within townships were given to the shack owners. My in-laws' address had no street name, just the symbol of the township zone next to the shack number. Having prepared to visit an exceptionally poor home, I was astonished to see their bungalow boasting a few bedrooms. Apparently, their shack had been extremely small in the apartheid era, with several children crammed inside their only room. However, by the time I visited them in 2004, as their children had grown up and started working, more rooms had been added. Water was a problem, hence each shack in the area had its own well, somehow intricately connected to their running water systems. I admired their clever running well water, and I admired all the things they had done on their own.

Eddie's dad was a self-taught handyman, and he had constructed or repaired most things around their home himself, sometimes with the family's help. There were DIY floors, very even and smooth. Eddie was concerned there were still some gaps under the roof of the house, although I enjoyed the sounds of the nocturnal insects that were clearly audible through those gaps as we slept at night. As in every other shack in their township, there were stylish bars in the windows and doors. While our Johannesburg neighbourhood was full of barbed wire on top of tall garden walls, Eddie's home township was full of window bars. Everyone was wary of crime.

***

We were all surprised to learn different things about each

other, both families learning different little details. I had brought a couple of glossy colourful books about Poland for my visit. We were seated in his parents' living room as his mother took time studying my book. There was a photo showing a large crowd of Poles kneeling at one Catholic pilgrimage centre before the revered painting of our Black Madonna of Częstochowa. The four old scars carved on Our Madonna's dark cheek now remind me of social media's hashtag symbol.

Eddie's mum paused over that photo. She was a devout Christian. Even though her Dutch Reformed Church had banned its black parishioners from attending white parishioners' services, Eddie's mum remained a regular churchgoer. She always attended her black community's services on Sundays, wearing her hat. I thought she was going to comment on the religious side of the photo in my book. She could not speak English, so the other family translated for us.

"Mum says those people are dressed rather poorly, perhaps," they said.

Her comment struck me. I had not looked at this photo that way, but indeed she was right.

"Yes," I said, "a lot of Poles are rather poor. You would see quite a lot of people dressed in a similar way."

"It is startling to see a country like yours," they replied. "Here, white people are mostly rich and black people are mostly poor, and it is strange to see so many poor whites at the same time. It is one thing to know a fact, but it is another thing to see with your own eyes. It is a strange feeling to see this picture."

"I don't think I am going to make my compote this year," my mum said to me in Poland later. "I can't believe I sweat here over my jars to make my own fruit compote for the winter, while Eddie's mum drinks her fancy juices from the cartons they buy."

"She would probably make her own compote, too, if they

had a different climate. And she does not have a lot of her own fruit."

"I know. I understand this. But then, she seems able to afford some things I cannot," Mum said.

Eddie's family's food was one of the things my mum had asked about, trying to learn and compare things. We usually had some spicy meat and white rice in South Africa. Eddie's father always had his maize meal instead, but I never had a chance to try that. Eddie told me it was not very tasty anyway. He told me rice was considered the side dish of the wealthier people, which is why he chose it whenever we went shopping. I noticed large packets of maize meal in supermarkets, but Eddie dissuaded me from trying the poorer staple food. The other day, when I reached for some packets of food in a shop, Eddie said this food gave out a strong smell while cooking. We returned it onto the shelf.

"You really don't want to cook it," he said.

My mum genuinely liked Eddie's mum from my stories, and I adored my mother-in-law. Eddie's mum was brave and clever. She had never been to school, but when her children had first gone to their schools, she had studied with them at home. She effectively taught herself to read. She was always keeping herself busy, just like my mum. She worked as a cleaner, but at home she either made or mended clothes; I remember her bent over her sewing machine.

Eddie's mum once told me I should sing whenever I feel lonely.

"You are far away from your home", she said. "You may feel sad. Sing if you feel lonely, and your music will accompany you."

***

During my stay in South Africa, there were things I was not allowed to do. One day I said we should go to the centre of Johannesburg before I left. I said we had not been there yet.

"Why would you want to do that?" asked one of Eddie's sisters.

Her question surprised me.

"I always go to city centres," I said, "It is nice to see the sights."

"Ah, no," they said, "there are no sights, we can tell you. There are immigrants from other African countries begging in the centre and it is dangerous. You could get stabbed. We can go to the cinema at the mall. We are not going to the city centre."

They also never agreed to my using the public transport. They have those minibuses that seem to have no fixed times of departure; at least, that was the case when I visited South Africa in 2004. I thought it could be fun sharing some of those local experiences by catching a minibus.

"No, you would always be the only white on any minibus you boarded", they said, and again they thought I would be everybody's most obvious target for any crime.

We only travelled by car and there was always a group of men as I travelled. Brother, cousin, uncle: always some men for my security, as the whole family were on red alert. They all felt their country was not a safe place for me and Eddie to be. Overall, his family were fabulous to me.

***

Some English words are different in South Africa. They say "robots" for traffic lights, or "rest shoes" for slippers, but most of all I remember the word, "sharp".

"Sharp!" Eddie greeted other black people there.

"Sharp!" they would say back.

They pronounced it more like "shup" and it meant either "hi" or "bye". I wondered how the word had originated as a greeting. Had it been about staying alert?

I felt I always had my best seat and my best view during my visit to Africa, because I had my best possible guide. Eddie knew a lot and he would explain various subtleties to me. Not every African knows several African languages, not even in South Africa with their eleven official languages. Most people speak just one African language, their own. Eddie spoke several of them and he liked to know about the different African cultures he sometimes spoke to me about.

One day, we visited a National Park to see some wild animals. A Welsh professional ranger drove us around. On our way, the ranger stopped his car and spoke to some black guards. He said something in an African language to the guards. They looked at him in silence until we drove away.

"They don't speak Tswana in this part of the country", said Eddie to the Welsh ranger.

The Welsh ranger did not understand.

"Tswana. You said those few words in this African language, in Tswana. Almost nobody speaks that language in this part of the country. Not to mention that I don't think those guards were South African at all. They did not understand you. It is best to speak English. At least, everyone will understand."

I was silent, but it occurred to me that it was ironic that our ranger, who was incredibly knowledgeable about his animals, seemed lost on seeing African faces; he seemed to be unaware that there existed more than one indigenous African language. He really was a good ranger, and I would strongly recommend him, however living in Africa he was unable to tell the local human differences, so he generally "spoke African" to all black Africans, regardless.

***

We were stopped twice by police cars during my stay in S.A. The police had received some phone calls about a white woman seen in a car with three black men, and assumed she was probably getting kidnapped. We were chased by two black police officers, who waited with us for two white police officers to arrive, and then we all waited for a plain-clothes white officer to close the case. I was shocked.

"Where are you from?" the Afrikaner policewoman asked me.

"I am from Europe," I replied.

She checked my passport.

"Ah, you are from Poland", she said, and she giggled.

I was fuming when they left.

"But you are not criticising them, are you?" asked Eddie. "Don't you criticise them. They did this for your sake. The truth is, there have been recent cases in this area of white women getting kidnapped, raped, and killed by groups of black men. They thought we were another case like that."

We also were followed by an off-road vehicle once, filled with armed para-military white men; Eddie told me later they had wanted to speak to me, so they must have said something in Afrikaans. Their vehicle stopped following us only after Eddie recorded them with his camera from the back of our car.

**

We were struggling to find a date for our wedding with any registrar in Johannesburg. Eddie told me that whenever he produced my documents with my photo, everyone realised they were fully booked. In the end, we got married nearby, in Alexandra. Eddie's cousin was my witness, and a random cabbie who drove us to Alexandra was Eddie's witness. The cabbie did not even seem surprised at being asked. I had to dip my fingertips in some black substance and leave my fingerprints on a document in the hall, and then we stood in a queue of casually dressed couples. Eddie told me most of the people would have arrived there straight from their work in the fields, for the formality of signing their marriage papers, and that everyone was planning their proper big African wedding for another day. Eddie and I were planning our proper wedding in Poland or in the UK, in church. Somebody in the queue spoke to Eddie and then gave me a dirty look. It was only much later that Eddie explained to me the man had asked Eddie to lend him the jacket of Eddie's suit for the man's ceremony.

"Why didn't you lend it to him then?" I asked.

"No way, he could have stained or damaged it. I told him you wouldn't have allowed it."

Suddenly I understood I had been right to think the man and his bride had been giving me hostile looks.

Our registrar was from the Pedi people, one of the black ethnic minority groups in South Africa. Eddie told me Pedi people followed ancient traditions, unfortunately including female genital mutilation. Eddie did not know if there was female genital mutilation in other local ethnic groups. During our wedding ceremony, the registrar mostly spoke in a language I did not understand. He then switched to English to ask me,

"Do you take Nkosiyabo Eduard Masondo as your lawfully wedded husband?"

Eddie later told me I had to forgive the registrar because he clearly did not speak enough English. I did not argue, but the registrar clearly had some English, because, at the end of our short ceremony he said to Eddie in English,

"Now keep earning your money."

Did the registrar think that, in 2004 in South Africa, the white bride must be a gold digger, and the black groom a rich man?

We celebrated with a nice lunch in a restaurant at the mall. I was happy we were married and about to start a new life together soon. I just had to wait for some time in the UK before Eddie could join me there. I did not know how long exactly it would take.

CHAPTER SEVEN – THE CLUBBER

"Please don't tell anyone we stayed here. Let's say we stayed at a nice hotel." Kama smiled.

She was seated opposite me on her bed, wearing her pyjamas, and brushing her long brown hair before sleep.

"Oh, definitely," I replied. "We stayed at a lovely hotel. We also met some utterly handsome guys at a nightclub as we went out clubbing."

She burst out into her giggly girly laughter.

We worked together in London at "Five Stars" the linen hire company, in telephone-based customer services around 2006. Kama was a new assistant in our team, and, because our manager was ever absent, I had been the one to give her some training on the job and to initially take over the more difficult calls from her. She was a delicate creature to me and a slightly crazy, fun, arty type. It was Kama who had suggested we travel somewhere together for a weekend, and I loved the spontaneity of this idea.

Having run to the departure gate we were the last two passengers to board our plane to Barcelona. We had not planned our trip well, but our spirits were high. Although it was only February, we soon left our winter jackets in a luggage locker in Barcelona's Nord bus station since the weather was lovely and warm. We got a hostel address from the information centre at the station; at the hostel we were given a strange room squashed behind a partition wall on the staircase landing. The room floor was covered with cold tiles, in black and white squares, like the staircase, and there were some noisy pipes running along the wall near our beds.

We both hated the room. Kama complained the sound of the water in the pipes near our headboards was making her want to pee. We laughed, but we left early in the morning for plenty of sightseeing through the day.

Like me, Kama was Polish. There were plenty of Poles working for Five Stars, perhaps because no English language skills were required in the laundry processing area, or perhaps because we were the people to snatch the minimum wage jobs. There were mostly women, a lot of them very pretty, and most of them worked with the speed and precision of machines.

Kama and I worked upstairs at the office with several other people. We took turns preparing lunch for our semi-retired financial controller Walter, due to his age. Walter was the only one in the business who was English born and bred. He sometimes joked over lunch about how one Ukrainian colleague had told him she was thrilled to meet a genuine Englishman at our London workplace. Walter praised our Bosnian accountant, Karima, for being perhaps the only person in the office to have a British sense of humour, or any sense of humour at all. To me, Walter was a distinguished gentleman living a successful life, although our boss Wasif remembered Walter getting picked on by some former colleagues in his younger days.

"I don't know if it was bullying, but perhaps some colleagues did not like him," Wasif said. "They once made a rag doll and attached it to the rear of his car, so Walter drove all the way to his home with that doll."

There was also Wesley, manager who had come to England from Jamaica as a five-year-old. Whereas I tried to help Kama during her first weeks on the job, it had been Wesley to go that extra mile for me during my first weeks, whenever his busy schedule allowed it. He had some advice for everyone.

Once, Karima was considering quitting: "Take a piece of

paper. On one side of the paper, write down everything you like about your job," he told her. "Then write on the other side why you want to leave and see which list is longer. Don't just make your decision without weighing things up."

"You now should learn one thing. You should learn to relax," was his advice to me.

Wesley had some fascinating stories to tell. He remembered a colonial map of the world he had seen in Jamaica, where Great Britain was a large island in the middle of the map as the rest of the world lay around this central island. Wesley said he had been impressed as a child at how big Great Britain looked compared to the rest of the world. I cannot blame him.

It was also Wesley who told me where the British two fingers offensive gesture had come from. It apparently harks back to the medieval English archers, whose index and middle fingers were essential for pulling the bow and therefore these two fingers were often chopped off in Norman captivity. Whoever had those fingers would stick them at their enemies in an intimidating gesture meaning "I can still shoot".

Wesley once took me along with him as he visited one client's restaurant in the City of London. He had notified me in advance so that I would have time to put on some smart clothes. As we walked toward the restaurant, he showed me around the area.

"All the biggest banks are here, '' Wesley was saying as we walked, "This is the heart of the financial City of London. Now see the people around. They are on their way to work, and they all look so sad!"

When I say Kama seemed a delicate creature, I mean she often seemed anxious, or nervous.

"I have discovered a very good use of mobile phones," she said to me once, "Do you ever feel tense and embarrassed in the street because you cannot help smiling or laughing for no reason? I sometimes do, and I have started checking my mobile phone or putting it against my ear when I pass by other people, so they do not stare at me for laughing to myself."

She was certainly creative in her neurotic survival skills.

Never in my life had I spent as much time clubbing as I did at Five Stars. Our Polish HR assistant Klaudia was looking for a husband in London nightclubs, and I often went clubbing with her. She would chat up various young men while I danced alone. Klaudia was in her early 20s, with blonde hair and a small shapely nose. The men in the clubs seemed happy for her to chat them up.

Klaudia sometimes helped at weekends at a launderette in West Hampstead, our district of London at the time. I accompanied her one Sunday afternoon. As she got busy serving some customers, I spread my newspaper out at the end of her counter, and I bent over my half-solved crossword.

"What crossword is this?" said one customer to me.

"Oh, it is just an easy one. I cannot do cryptic." I smiled.

"You are doing an English crossword. I haven't seen that here before."

The customer spoke to Klaudia about his change.

"You know I wouldn't overcharge you," she smiled.

"I actually think you could," replied the man. "You probably would overcharge me." Then he turned to me.

"And you wouldn't," he said to me, before leaving the shop.

I felt awkward after he left. Klaudia had previously tended to work with livestock on some farms abroad as a teenager, and I thought she had had to toughen up. Some people may have perceived her as harsh. Unlike fragile Kama, Klaudia never had a problem smiling for no reason in the street. Klaudia was stable and solid, perhaps also crude, since she lifted once a Scotsman's kilt in my presence.

Klaudia did not want to return to her previous life on the farms. She had resolved to marry one of the men we could see in London nightclubs.

"I like the guys in nice shirts at the clubs," she said. "A lot of them tell me they are managers or accountants."

She regularly attended nightclubs for husband-hunting, and I was delighted to have that excuse for going out together. I loved the music, the lighting, and the crowds. I danced alone for most of the nights.

We were sometimes joined by other colleagues during our nights out.

"Is it true you're gay?" an English man asked me one day, at Cricklewood's "The Crown" hotel bar. I looked up as he continued, "Your friend told me she's gay and that you are her girlfriend. She is over there. Is that true?"

The man pointed towards our beautiful Kama. Like Klaudia, Kama was also in her 20s, also with a pretty face, and I thought she had the best figure of us all. While Klaudia was chubby and I saw myself as too skinny, Kama's body was the shape of an hourglass.

"Yes, it's true," I lied to the man. Kama swiftly joined us and as we hugged each other, I was hoping to look convincing.

Even Wesley joined us one night. He normally wore his suit at work, so it was fun seeing him wear an almost entirely open shirt at the club. He had a good chest.

***

When I was 15 years old, in 1988, I signed up for a short course in ballroom and Latin dancing. During one of those dance lessons, one girl exclaimed her partner had stepped on her toe.

"It was your fault he stepped on your toe", the female instructor interrupted straightaway. "You had taken his space. He is trying to lead, let him lead. To be honest, in this sort of dance, he is the leader, and you are only the decoration." The instructor had spoken bluntly to the girl, and I did not like her wording. One thing was for sure, I knew I was never going to be anybody's decoration in my whole life. I was confident that I was very much going to be my own person, and I thought our dance teacher had just demonstrated a disastrous choice of words. But then, she also showed us a rather special practical skill that she had.

"Now you are dancing with me, and I want you to try and step on my toe," she said to the boy.

I think it was more than one boy who later tried to step on her toe, but no-one could. She hovered over the dance floor with those boys – she had a very fit body, and she leaned back a bit. She looked elegant and totally effortless as the boys made their smaller and bigger steps, or slower and quicker steps, some of those steps clearly aimed at her foot no-one could step on.

"Can you see?" she said to us girls as they spun round the dance floor. "I am leveraging the arms lock, and I am making my steps a split second after his."

Well, I still did not want to be anybody's decoration in my life, although I certainly wanted to learn the same skill that she showed, and I did my best to never let anyone step on my toes when dancing.

There was a boy at my dance course who I heard some girls talking about. He seemed to only have vision in one eye, and he had rather average looks, but he danced like an angel, they said. The girls loved to waltz with him. I recognised him after dancing a few steps together. I enjoyed every kind of dance with him. We were probably over-expressive with our Spanish paso doble, for our feet stomping was loud and our head turns were sharp; as we played with and enjoyed that dance, our instructor looked at our pair and laughed. I loved moving to music. And now, 20 years later in London, I felt happiest with the lights dimmed and the rhythmical tunes loud. I spent lots of time on the dancefloor.

***

Clubbing was the core of my private life. The truth was, I simply did not have much private life outside regular phone calls from Eddie, who still lived away from the UK. While Klaudia attended clubs to chase her dreams, I went there to escape my otherwise lonely evenings. There were people having fun, and I cherished their presence around me, and I soaked in the joy of those nights with my every cell, to charge my entire weekend with this positive feeling.

CHAPTER EIGHT – THE GRASS WIDOW

I lived on my own in 2005 and 2006, although formally I was married. I thought my life was ultimately screwed up that way. My new husband Eddie had taken a new job in an American corporation away from me. He had never asked my opinion when applying for a job overseas from me, and I felt disappointed and angry at him. I had spent a couple of years renting a double accommodation in London, a requirement for me to apply for Eddie's spousal visa, although I was not earning much. My initial employment terms with Five Stars the laundry were 37.5 hours per week at £4.85 per hour. £9,457.50 per annum as of late 2004, and nearly all my money was spent on my home that I was keeping ready for Eddie. Higher-earning Eddie spent years planning to join me in the UK at some unspecified time when his career plans allowed it. Some of Eddie's colleagues told him having a wife overseas was not a real marriage.

"I told them our love was above sex," Eddie said to me.

I was not enthusiastic about hearing that, although I somehow felt too embarrassed to protest. Then I finally said I wanted a divorce.

"I do not want to be divorced!" Eddie exclaimed, and I always felt that was the truest expression of how he felt. He had spent years building his life according to his grand plans. Being married was part of his plans, however dysfunctional our lives became, and he saw divorce as failure. He wanted me to continue waiting for him.

***

The Lower Ground Bar in West Hampstead, North-west London, has been described online as somewhere "you did not want to be seen leaving after a night out". Since I was living opposite it, in West End Lane, the club was convenient for me though, and I often hung out there. The bar may have been a bit scruffy, with a small dancefloor, but I liked most of the music, and the atmosphere was fun late at night. One evening in 2006, one year before my first mental breakdown, I stood alone with a glass of whisky and Coke in the Lower Ground Bar. The loudspeakers were pouring out a thudding techno tune as I waited for some other rhythms, for those more uneven ones, like the rhythm of a heartbeat: perhaps for my favourite R'n'B hits of the year.

"You look a bit lost," a male voice said to my ear.

I turned to see a pleasant-looking man whose hair was shining golden in the club lights. Klaudia, who I had come out with, was away chatting to some men, while indeed I was just waiting beside the dancefloor on my own. I smiled at the man as he was right: I was feeling awkward among the crowd of strangers.

"What do you do?" he asked.

"Oh no, let's not talk about jobs," I said.

"Why not? What do you do?"

"OK then, I work on the phone, but I don't like my job. I don't want to talk about what I do", I replied, perhaps abruptly.

I thought he would walk away, however he did not. He paused and gave me a lingering look.

"Some nice little sex line, perhaps?" he said with a cheeky smile.

To my own surprise, this question broke the ice, as something inside me melted. This man with his posh English accent and peculiar demeanour reminded me of the "*Bridget Jones's Diary*" movie scene where the main heroine gets introduced as one who "played in his fountain naked". (She had done as a baby.) I suddenly wanted to be outrageous, too.

"I was once tempted to," I admitted.

"How do you mean?"

"I was really struggling with my job search when I first arrived in London, and in those jobs, they were always looking for new staff," I replied. "So, I remember myself hungry and pondering over a newspaper ad that was recruiting females for a sex phone line."

"And?... How did it end? Did you apply?"

"No, I did not," I concluded, and I was given a brightest smile.

"So, what do you do?" I asked, assuming it was something he wanted to talk about.

He was an arm surgeon, and he had come to the club with another doctor, a psychiatrist.

"He is very Freudian," was his comment about his psychiatrist friend, and he made me laugh. It was happy laughter. None of my colleagues in my first years in London had ever mentioned psychology, and my colleagues were all I had known here. This new surgeon seemed as if he was from a different world, and he reminded me of my own young days spent over books.

"I work for a laundry," I explained. "There is nothing wrong with my job really, except I would prefer something with more meaning to it."

"All right then, let me rephrase it. What would you like to do?"

"I don't know. I used to be a schoolteacher in Poland."

"You should teach here. We need teachers in England."

"It is not that straightforward," I protested. "I sometimes struggle to understand some people here. It would be a disaster if I could not understand my own pupils. You've got to have the connection."

The arm surgeon asked me to excuse him and disappeared in the crowd. He reappeared with a small glass of vodka for me.

"I cannot drink vodka straight – I am not used to it," I explained. I felt the man seemed disappointed though, so I took the vodka off him, and we mixed it with my other drink.

"You are not Polish if you cannot drink vodka," he murmured.

"And you are not a doctor if you have me up my drinks," I replied between my sips.

The psychiatrist came over to see if the surgeon was doing alright.

"I have met a few people. They're over there. Do come over and meet them too," the psychiatrist said to his friend.

The surgeon introduced me to the psychiatrist, saying I was Polish.

"Cześć", the psychiatrist said hi in Polish to me, and he added in English, "I like vodka."

They disappeared together, though I later noticed the surgeon near the wall, slumped on a chair on his own. He looked sad. I felt sorry for him and came over asking him to dance.

"They have stolen my jacket," he said, "I left my leather jacket here."

He got up to dance though. He held my waist saying I was probably part of the mafia who had robbed him.

"You must have been a very good teacher," he said after a while, to my surprise. "There is something about your personality that makes me feel you were."

***

In September 1995, my 15-year-old male pupils were new to their school, and they still seemed shy in their new surroundings. During one of my first lessons with them, I heard them murmur behind my back that I had made an English spelling mistake on the blackboard. Or maybe it was the wrong month in the date at the top. I simply remember myself pausing to look at what I had written, and indeed there was an error on the blackboard.

"Who said I wrote that wrong?" I asked, turning toward the group. There was silence in the classroom. Nobody wanted to argue with me.

"No-one?"

One generally cheeky boy, Krzyś, slowly raised his hand, leaning back in his chair, his legs spread casually.

"I say you wrote that wrong," he said.

"And what should I have written?" I asked again.

Krzyś corrected my mistake, explaining what I should have written.

"Excellent," I admitted, and I put down a top grade against his name in the register, which was lying open on my desk. This started an avalanche of other voices.

"I also said you had made a mistake," said another boy.

"And I said that, too. More of us noticed."

"I did ask my question a while ago, and you then had your opportunity to reply," I said. I ignored the other boys and only brave Krzyś scored in my class on that day.

I may have not been a typical teacher in that school, because I liked my pupils to be vocal rather than quiet. Better loud than silent, I thought. It was nice for me to hear in 2006 that somebody believed I may have been good.

***

"How about we have a nice dinner one day?" the arm surgeon asked. "I will not buy you vodka this time. I would get you some nice wine you could savour. What do you say?"

I hesitated. A part of me wanted to see him again, but I declined his invitation.

"Why not?" he asked, "Do you have a husband and children waiting for you at home?"

"I have no children."

"Husband?" He looked me in the eye.

"I have a husband overseas," I said.

"And what now? Separation?"

"I don't know what next. I honestly do not know."

We bid goodbye as they were closing the club in early morning.

"There's your friend coming over," said Klaudia to me as we stood on the pavement outside the club, waiting for somebody she had been talking to.

The psychiatrist was leaving with some stunning giggling women, and he kept telling the surgeon to keep up with them. I looked nothing like those women. Tall and slender with proportionate facial features, they could be models.

I thought it was nice that the surgeon found the time to come over to me and ask if I was fine going home. I said I was, and I showed him one of the West End Lane buildings opposite us, where I was renting my place.

Then he waved goodbye to me from the window of their black cab and disappeared from my life.

His question, "What now," stayed with me though.

CHAPTER NINE – THE SCANDALIST

Now that I am a post-psychotic person, I notice how they use the word "psychotic" in the movies. They sometimes say things like, "him and his psychotic girlfriend," although there is no mention of the girlfriend having mental health difficulties, or "oh, her father is a totally psychotic type, a real killer". I don't think psychotic is a personality trait, so I believe people often confuse the words "psychotic" and "psychopath", as if these two words meant the same thing. I don't consider myself a psychopath, but then I do have some embarrassing memories of myself, so judge for yourself and do read on.

***

In the summer of 2006, I left the double accommodation I had been keeping for Eddie for two years. I moved into a single room overlooking some rose bushes, their sweet scent lingering lazily in the summer air. Fresh-smelling linen was made ready on my bed for me, and a small soft toy rested on the mantelpiece. The room felt old-fashioned in a calming way; it looked exactly how I would imagine a granny's spare room. There was a live-in landlady who I never saw get out of her room, and her son, a silver-haired Englishman called Hugh, who was extremely proud of their house, which had retained all its original features from around the time of the war. They certainly had some historic electric meters in that house – ones operated by old British shillings. Hugh kept plenty of old shillings, which he sold to us tenants so we could operate the electric meters. Then he recycled those coins by emptying the meters and by selling us those shillings again in return for our contemporary British pounds. He rented out several of their bedrooms to females only, and prior to renting a room he held interviews with short-listed female candidates to make sure we all fitted in. All us girls in that house were slim, with medium to long hair, and each arrived at Hugh's place being single. I guess we all were between 25 and 35 years old. Hugh was over 60 and he held his weekly meetings with each tenant.

"Will you find some time for a chat with an old man?" he would ask.

He always had his cider ready for our meetings in his living room and each day of his week was devoted to a different tenant. I think mine were Tuesdays.

Hugh told me about his other tenants during our meetings. An English girl lived in the attic whose new boyfriend later started sleeping overnight in her room. The English girl had apparently told Hugh directly never to touch her possessions and Hugh told me she was therefore "very odd".

There was a gregarious Irish girl with an utterly charming air about her. I shared a kitchen with her, and I liked her from the start. She was surrounded by friends, and Hugh must have liked her too, because he confessed to me that he had suggested to her the two of them should get together. He said she had even joked to him about condoms but had grown very distant afterwards. He asked my opinion, and I tried to delicately dissuade him from pursuing it any further.

Then there was a stunning German girl. I had always admired the German model, Claudia Schiffer, and Hugh's German tenant was almost as gorgeous, to me. She soon started dating a young man though, and Hugh bitterly told me, "The men up at the pub would describe women like her in their own way." There was a Thai girl who also started dating very soon but who held long conversations with Hugh about his fetishes, he said. Apparently, she even suggested different websites where he was to look for his like-minded playmates. Finally, there was me. Hugh told me he had always liked my legs, and the fact I had been married, which he thought meant I was familiar with "men and their desires", as he put it. Hugh was apparently interested in what he called "corrective therapy", or sessions of naked spanking. I had an uneasy feeling he was hoping for me to join in, but I did not say much.

"One girl is about to move out," he told me one Tuesday, "and I normally perform certain rituals in a former tenant's room, to get rid of the bad vibes. Do you mind?"

I said I did not mind.

"I also tend to be naked at the time," he continued. "Do you mind?"

Unsurprisingly, I moved out of Hugh's as soon as I could, to rent a bedsit in Harlesden with a live-out landlord.

***

Gradually, Five Stars saw some potential in me and by 2007 I was already earning £20,000 per annum there, more than twice my initial minimum wage. Earlier though, in 2005 and 2006 I could just about afford to go clubbing once a week. Klaudia and I often entered the clubs early enough to walk in free. Sometimes, women had free entry throughout the night. I bought a couple of drinks per night and that was my budget used up. However, being a lonely "grass widow" for a couple of years, with no husband by my side but also with no children to cherish, weighed me down. I also felt frustrated because, as I went to clubs, there were always some men interested in dating, and I would have loved to date someone again, yet I felt tied by my formal marriage to my ever-absent spouse. In the end, my loneliness got the better of me. I am not proud of myself, but the reality is, I finally decided to find someone for sex, most likely for my first ever one-night stand.

I created a profile with an online dating site called Match.com. It was heavily advertised and there were lots of user profiles. Paul was my online choice. He seemed to be local to London. I wanted a local man; someone who was present there in the flesh. I looked for somebody with a degree first. I was aware many people with no formal education are brilliant and wise, but having a choice online, I tried to find someone who might be more studious. Paul was divorced, taller than I, had a university degree, liked the gym, and something about him made me feel that he had no desire for instant commitment. I liked all of that. I chatted him up, or should I say I wrote first, and we met for a date. We went for a long walk together. Paul looked streetwise and he called me "a snob", for not wanting to sit together on a wall by the pavement. It was only much later that I saw him wear the formal suit that was required for his workplace. I found him witty and down-to-earth.

I lured Paul to my place with some dessert the second time we met. After some polite conversation I got my first kiss and everything else that I wanted. We first had sex that afternoon. My plan seemed to be working well. Before my first cosy evening with Paul, I had seen lots of attractive men in clubs, but when I went clubbing after my first evening with him, I only saw average men. My sexual frustration seemed to have left me. On the other hand, perhaps my initial plan never quite worked as I never really had a one-night stand with Paul. Instead, we kept coming back to each other. We went to the cinema together and he bought me a copy of a book he loved. We talked about lots of things. He was an attentive listener and an honest critic, and I genuinely loved every moment of talking together. I sketched Paul's portrait in my notebook once after he fell asleep at my place. His face looked chiselled with some strong straight lines. He told me, and wrote to me by email, some nice things about me. He was the first person ever to use the lovely English word, "integrity", to describe me. He thought I had integrity, and, once I looked up the word in an online dictionary, I loved the comment. I kept all his emails in my inbox to read them over and over.

"So, your date is British? Does he have a sexy English accent?" asked Andrea, my Hungarian colleague at Five Stars. "I love English accents. If I had an English boyfriend, I would have him speak to me constantly. Only speak. I would get high by listening."

I invited Paul to one event I was going to with my colleagues, but he declined.

"Perhaps another time," he said.

I was probably in love with Paul by the time he sent me an email saying, "I like you, but I am not in love with you" – and then things faded, and we later stopped seeing each other. I kept all his sweet earlier emails though.

***

I already considered myself separated when I once met Eddie in west London to talk. I hoped the two of us could part as friends. Eddie snatched my mobile phone from my hand to move my SIM card from my old phone into a new, better handset that he gave me instead. He said it was his present for me. I thought it was a lovely surprise gift. I never thought much about Eddie keeping my old handset, which he said he needed as his own replacement phone.

He later continued to phone me from abroad and warned me against ignoring his calls. He said he would phone my colleagues' phone numbers that he had found on my old mobile handset. I spent many months trying to appease Eddie and to make sure I would answer his every phone call. In 2007, I phoned my local police station.

"My estranged husband is making threats to me that he is going to harass my work colleagues," I complained.

The woman who took my call told me to calm down.

"He has not really done anything," she replied.

The blackmail went on for months and I remained available for Eddie's calls all those months, until one day when I left my phone at home overnight as I went clubbing. Eddie phoned Klaudia's mobile in the small hours of that night.

"I don't want to be receiving any more phone calls from Eddie!" shouted Klaudia at me at the door of our office on Monday morning.

"Klaudia, I can go to the police with you..." I suggested.

"But I don't want to go to the police!"

"I'll pay for your phone if you would like to change your number."

"I don't want to change my number! Do you understand me? I have no intention of changing it! I just want to stop receiving his calls!"

I was convinced that everyone at Five Stars, even silently, blamed me for Eddie's behaviour. I felt acutely ashamed of my poor choice of husband and of the fact I had not been able to protect my colleagues. Our Five Stars office phone line started getting jammed by my estranged husband, who called repeatedly; my colleagues just kept on putting their receivers down in silence. I so wanted to disappear somewhere within the big city. So, I browsed job ads in my local newspaper and at the job centre.

CHAPTER TEN – THE RUNAWAY

I was surprised to lose access to my private email in 2007. My password had been changed. My colleagues, ex-colleagues, ex-pupils, and my family started receiving some disturbing sexualised emails from my address. I first learnt from my family about this.

"Do not worry about it," Radek said to me over the phone, "Nobody who knows you will ever believe it was you writing all that."

I suspected Eddie, especially as the nasty emails were often about me being unfaithful to Eddie. Clearly the person who had accessed my inbox showed a particular interest in Paul's earlier complimentary emails I had kept.

"I don't think your email was hacked," said Wesley after I told him it had been. "It was probably accessed by someone close to you who knew your old password or your security question. Never select a password that is meaningful to you. Select something abstract. For example, 'parrot'."

For a long time, my password subsequently was: "Wesleysparrot".

Wesley never told me they had received any of those emails at work. One day, on my arrival at Five Stars' office, all my colleagues suddenly went silent. I had a terrible apprehension that something bad was about to surface, and I could not stop feeling scared. Finally, Wasif called me to a different room for a chat.

"I believe you should know that there are some emails coming to the office about you," he said.

It turned out that pretty much everyone at the office

apart from me had received those emails in their individual inboxes. I was thoroughly ashamed. I thanked Wasif for telling me, and I was truly grateful for that, but I felt shattered. After that, I started my every day with a feeling of deep embarrassment and my shame was never gone. Every morning was spent wondering what my colleagues would find in their mailboxes on their arrival. I tried my best to keep my workload unaffected.

"We have received some emails saying your husband's passed away," Wasif said another day to me in his office.

"Has he again?" I only said. My sister had received similar news on her phone weeks before, which had then proved to be untrue. I felt completely numb.

"That's what I thought," Wasif concluded, "I will not trouble you again about these emails."

Ever since Wasif showed me an example of those incoming emails, I had been worrying about Paul. Paul's email address was constantly being mentioned in Eddie's emails and I was scared Eddie might finally manage to hack Paul's account as well. I started feeling intensely afraid that Paul might have to go through the same hell as me, with all workplace emails bombarded by hostile communications. I texted Paul's phone to warn him.

"I will not delete my email address," he texted back, "I will be fine. Don't worry about me."

I continued to worry, nonetheless.

***

I took up a part-time job as a receptionist at a GP surgery in Queens Park in spring 2007. It was part of my effort to gradually change jobs and to disappear from my estranged husband's view.

My position at the GP reception was a minimum wage job and I only worked in the mornings. In those days, I did not know people on low income could top up their wages with welfare in the UK. I did not even know whether I was eligible for any welfare, even though both Poland and the United Kingdom were in the European Union at the time. I worried that perhaps in this country my estranged husband might need to apply for benefits with me if I was formally married. I really was a mess – it simply never occurred to me I should research what help I was eligible for. I had always worked since finishing school, and all I wanted to do was continue working. I started looking for one more new job for my afternoons, and meanwhile I was trying to learn as much as I could about the GP surgery I was working for.

***

I was delighted to finally be part of an organisation that served the British public. Back at Five Stars, I had also sometimes experienced the wonderful feeling of being useful to others, though it had been more about helping specific businesses rather than the public. At the GP Surgery, it would no longer be other businesses I would assist. Instead, I would deal with individuals in need. I liked that. I was proud that our doctor was doing a crucial job, and I was happy to be helping. On the other hand, not everything was easy at our surgery. One difficulty was that our boss, the doctor, frequently shouted either at his patients, or at his non-medical staff.

"Why do you never cry when the doctor shouts at you?" asked Vesna, our medical secretary from Serbia, "When I started working here, I cried a lot."

I liked Vesna, although it did not sound right to me anyone should cry at work to appease their bosses. Anyway, I never cried because I was too proud to do so. I just swallowed all the insults in silence, as I had always done my whole life.

"Did you type something in this patient's file on your computer?!" the doctor yelled at me one day in front of some patients at the reception, "Somebody entered wrong details in her file after I last saw her, and it must have been you, because you don't know anything, and you think you do!"

He pointed at some abbreviation of a medical term in her

file that we looked up on my computer. I did not know what the abbreviation stood for.

"I wonder who knows such difficult words as this one," I said, trying to be politely diplomatic without directly pointing at my boss.

The doctor went silent.

"Forget it. I wrote it," he said quickly and disappeared in his consulting room.

Years later, that surgery was closed by the local council as "inadequate" and for posing a "threat to its patients". I learnt about it from local news online. I also read some online reviews by former staff and patients that mentioned "a lack of privacy", or described our doctor as "sexist, racist, speaks about his staff in derogatory terms".

No-one seemed responsible for keeping things organised. A nurse told us at the reception during the break that some of our vaccines were out of date. Nobody at the reception seemed to oversee monitoring the supplies. Nobody at all seemed to be in charge of anything, apart from the doctor. The patients were seen in no particular order, depending on the doctor's preference, and I had difficulty explaining to some patients why they were kept waiting an hour past their planned appointment time. One patient's file disappeared after a consultation. The doctor yelled at us, the receptionists, as we searched high and low for a potentially misplaced file.

***

I regularly checked for ads, searching for a second part-time job for myself. My local job centre finally advertised for a part-time data processing assistant for the afternoons. A jewel of a job, I reckoned. It seemed a splendid opportunity for me to fill my afternoons and to patch up my budget, which was strained by my poorly paid part-time morning job.

The recruitment process saw a group of us candidates sit together in a meeting room and take a mathematics test in writing. There was no interview and nearly no talk, although we were briefly told not to stress. I had always loved maths, and the young man who held the entrance test with us must have liked my results, because I got the job. The name in his email address was Nathan Meadowbank. I received his brief email inviting me straight to my first shift. I was to be a part-time Data Validation Assistant on the minimum wage. Fortunately, no expensive dress code was required.

The day before the start of my new afternoon job, my probation with the GP surgery came to an end. I was excitedly looking forward to signing my permanent contract for my reception job while starting my data validation job, too. Things may have not been ideal, but I felt happy and hopeful. I seemed to be finding my feet in my quest to escape my hapless recent past.

At the end of my shift, the doctor asked me to his consulting room. The conversation, however, was not what I had expected.

"You are clean and honest," he said, "but I don't think we work well together. This has been your last day of your probation, and I will not sign an employment contract with you. I will not be needing you tomorrow morning."

I was shocked. Having left home in the morning an employed person, I was returning in the afternoon unemployed. For the first time somebody had given up on me at work, something I had not anticipated, and I was shaken. I was also running out of time trying to secure myself enough hours at a job Eddie would not know about, before I ran out of my meagre savings.

***

Clever Costs was nested in a spacious, bright open-plan office above some shops in Edgware Road in 2007. There were rows of identical desks with computer monitors sitting on the tight rows of desks. Staff did not keep any personal objects at their workstations. You did not have a permanent desk; you were expected to move seats instead. This is what

Nathan Meadowbank, who had handled my recruitment process, explained to me on my arrival. I would now call it "hot-desking", although I was never shown where to book a desk of my choice in advance if I wanted to sit next to specific people, as they do in so many other offices nowadays.

The list of company policies that Nathan had emailed to me before my first day said there was no specific dress code in the office, although I had seen during my recruitment process that the staff looked neat and professional. The boys wore formal shirts. Perhaps they enjoyed working within an office setting and preferred traditional long sleeve shirts over casual T-shirts. The girls wore smart dresses or some nice tops at their desks, and I was wearing my hippie beads with my best clothes for my first shift. I really wanted to be there.

I worried over my timing, as the clock on my computer was not set properly, and my first shift was to last three hours only. I was somehow ashamed to tell anyone I had forgotten to take my phone or my watch from home, so I had no time-measuring device whatsoever. I had lost my receptionist's job just the day before, and since my previous boss, the doctor, had told me I was difficult for him to work with, I was desperately nervous at Clever Costs, planning to be as humble, meek and quiet as possible. I was feeling scared.

I was not introduced to anyone at the start of my first shift. They had already been seated at their desks on my arrival, so I quietly perched at a desk Nathan Meadowbank chose for my first shift for me. Wanting to do well, I ferociously focused on my new workload as per instructions from… the King of Spades. Let me explain.

***

Back at my family home, my Granny sometimes pretended to be reading her playing cards for us, for some fortune-telling fun. Different cards carried different meanings. The nine and ten of Clubs stood for trouble. The nine and ten of Spades stood for health matters. The Diamonds stood for money, and the Ace of Diamonds was a letter. The Hearts, of course, stood for love, and aces coming together stood for change. King, Queen, and Jack of Spades stood for friends. Senior Hearts stood either for friends, or for older people. Senior Clubs stood either for enemies, or for some officials. I excitedly watched Gran unfold her cards, like a kaleidoscope of little mysteries, even though she always warned us not to take any of it seriously.

I never had a chance to learn the names of most colleagues at Clever Costs, therefore I gave them the card names for the sake of my memoir. The King of Spades represented someone friendly. The man who briefly trained me on my job seemed amiable too. I am not sure he ever told me his name, or if he did, I don't remember it, hence I invented this nickname for him. My King of Spades. He looked Asian, with fantastically thick black hair and dark eyes behind his glasses. He worked with his earphones on. Though, he seemed to be everyone's friend.

***

One young woman walked over to my desk and crouched next to my chair.

"Cześć. Jesteś Polką? – Hi. Are you Polish?" she whispered in Polish to me. "Nathan told me. I am Polish too, and he thought we could become good friends. My name is Nina." She gave me a discreet handshake under the level of my desk.

"Nathan is not a real manager", she continued whispering in Polish as no-one near us understood. "The managers are on holiday, and they asked him to do them a favour and take care of the recruitment. This is not his job. I am not even sure if he is getting paid for this. I would be surprised if he was. I feel for him," Nina looked at Nathan, then at me again. "More of us here are Polish. Will you join me for lunch so we can chat?"

As I gave all my colleagues the identities of cards, she

was my whispering Queen of Spades, or a secret spy in that Edgware Road office who passed information to me in Polish. I happily whispered back promising to go out to lunch together, but my short shift ended soon, and I never saw her again.

"How am I doing with the targets? the Queen of Clubs said to the King of Spades, "You can tell." The Queen of Clubs got up from her seat and walked over to lean over him. She had shiny long dark hair with a slightly tanned complexion and a foreign accent. I thought the Queen of Clubs might be from somewhere as distant as Latin America for instance.

"You are doing 78% of the target," the King of Spades said.

Like mine, her work must have been based within their in-house software. Some of us input data which others validated. Our work resembled a production line within an office setting. Clearly, the King of Spades must have been able to check the performance of each workstation in the network.

"Oh, really? And what about me? How am I doing?" asked somebody else.

A group of slender silhouettes gathered round the King of Spades who said, "You are doing 86%..." "You are doing 82%..."

"And how is she doing?", asked the menacing Queen of Clubs.

"Who?" replied King of Spades.

"She", repeated Clubs. "SHE." Who did she mean?

King of Spades gave in.

"She is doing 98%", he said.

"Why, this is only because she is not talking to anyone! She is horrible," concluded the Queen of Clubs.

When everybody got back to their seats, I walked over to the King of Spades.

"Can I also ask how I am doing?" I asked. My body felt

stiff, and I was desperately hoping the answer would not be 98%.

"You are doing 98%. This is before your work gets checked for any errors, when the percentage may go down," he said.

It dawned on me I was probably the "She".

Not everybody spoke about the mysterious "she", I am happy to say. Nathan told his colleagues a handful of interesting facts about himself on that day during my shift, and he got me hooked on listening. Nathan's voice, in that messy office, quickly became my lighthouse that kept me from despairing over the "She", over the doctor and over Eddie. At least I could focus on Nathan instead. He seemed to have told them certain things for the first time, like the fact that he had played bridge at his college, or that he sometimes visited his dad in the country. Some people next to him seemed not to have known this. Since I was a small-town Pole, I would have loved to hear more about what life had been like in Nathan's dad's town or village in the English countryside. I had never been anywhere in the UK outside London. I knew I had been eavesdropping, stealing all that information without connecting somehow, but I was hoping to hear more from him.

***

In my college days back in Poland, I had once gate-crashed a private party held on St Andrew's Day on the ground floor of the students' hotel that I lived in. St Andrew's Day on 30th November is traditionally party time in Poland. They organise dances. We even do our fortune-telling on that occasion, in most family homes. It was some Polish students of German language and literature who had organised the dance party in my hotel. Anybody from outside their German Studies group was supposed to pay for their entrance. The party was, however, gate-crashed by lots of students from the large building who arrived in crowds that included me. As we sat down inside, on chairs people had found or brought along, and our own bottles in front of us on the tables along the walls, I noticed one male German language student trying to check people's tickets. He raised his voice, sending one embarrassed blonde girl out the door. That, in turn, started a commotion because one of the sports students accused the German student of mistreating the woman.

"And what about you?" asked him the German language student, "Where is your ticket?"

I recognised the mouthy sports student. I had once played a game of rubber bridge against him. The two of us were in the minority of the hotel's residents who played the game. I did not want him to be kicked out of that party; otherwise, I would not mind getting kicked out with him.

"That's OK, he's here with me!" I shouted toward the German student from my table.

To this day, I do not know why the German language student never checked my non-existent ticket. I suppose he must have felt tired of us at that point. The mouthy bridge-loving student quickly caught on. He walked towards me and put his hands on my shoulders. We both looked at the German student.

"Really???" asked me the German language student venomously. "Keep him now in check then!"

That was one of my best parties of my lifetime to that date, because the gobby bridge-loving sports student introduced me that night as his "girlfriend" to probably every friend of his, and there were many, so I suddenly had plenty of men asking me to dance, and I loved it.

***

This is why, when Nathan said he had played bridge at college, it felt like accidentally finding a lump of gold. Nathan wasn't talking to me, but he did to other colleagues, and he was within an audible distance, so I kept on listening. I might have been his most avid listener, though I never commented on anything he said. He was my favourite radio station at that place. It was probably from that moment on that Nathan could do no wrong to me. In a way, he felt completely different to me when I compared him to the rest of the office; he felt a bit like a newly found cousin, or someone belonging in my own college world.

The painful thing was, he had no idea, because I never said anything. I was strangely unable to speak because that office paralysed me. I felt as if I was never going to be able to connect. For the first time in my life, I started feeling a bit disabled, psychologically, and perhaps I already was. I mean that topic was one I wanted to engage with, but I failed, at that desperately lonely point of my life, even though it would have meant the world to me. Nobody else replied to Nathan about bridge, either. Perhaps nobody else had played bridge at college. I so much wanted that topic to go on; I wanted it to roll on gathering size like a snowball. However, the topic was dropped, so that one tantalising colourful balloon burst for me.

CHAPTER ELEVEN – THE RAINMAKER

"She used to be a teacher," said the Jack of Clubs to the other young male next to him at Clever Costs on my second day. "Would you like a teacher like that?"

***

"Engliiiiiish!" – some drunken male voices were shouting further down the street in Poland. I had just started teaching the English language at one technical school and that is how I know it must have been 1995, when I was 22. I was returning home from a night out. It was not a long walk back home, perhaps 15 minutes or less. I was wearing a mini skirt, and it seemed I had been recognised as a new teacher by that group of drunken young men. My own pupils never bothered me in the streets; they would not have dared, but I also think they simply would not have wanted to. This drunken group were either some of the oldest pupils at my school, or most probably they were no longer at school, but they still chose to see me as a teacher.

"Angielski!" they shouted in Polish; this means, "English!" Then they went on, "Will you fuck?"

I hated that label I had from my young age, that "teacher" thing. The worst part was not my job as such. I liked my classroom job. But wherever I went after work, in my small town, everybody knew who I was.

"Is that one of your pupils? The one sitting at the bar?"

asked Kira, my art school friend, at a club one night. "He has just hidden his cigarette on seeing you."

Smoking was still allowed in pubs and clubs in Poland at the time.

"No, he must be studying at my school though", I said. "He may be a minor if he hides his cigarette."

How could one enjoy clubbing while being watched so closely?

"Who was that man you were squeezing at the concert last weekend?" asked a fellow teacher at work, "The boys have told me they saw you."

"Ah, that would have been a boy from my school times, an old friend," I replied. "I never squeezed him, we leaned against each other's backs as we gazed at the stars. The boys are being silly."

I did not seem to have a private life anymore though. I suddenly turned old at 22, as a teacher in my small Polish town, and I hated that.

I started feeling young again after I came to London at 30. The foremost reason was that nobody knew me here and my new anonymous life felt liberating to me. Secondly, the clubbers in London were ageless. There were always people of all ages in London clubs, and I felt young again. I felt I belonged. I fell passionately in love with this city, and I clung to it. Even during my problems in 2007, I did not want to live anywhere else, I only wanted to hide within London. I was lucky to be starting a new job, however few hours I had initially been offered. If only I could now relax at my new office.

***

"I don't understand," said a white woman with blonde hair, a pointy nose and a British accent into the office space around us, apparently to no-one, on my second afternoon at Clever Costs. I shall call her the Queen of Hearts. "I don't understand what you were talking about. She is only a bit shy, that's all!"

My Queen of Hearts, seated next to me at the start of my second shift, had some empathy. If she was speaking about me, she was correct: I was being shy. Unfortunately, she was just leaving the office for the end of her shift, and I stayed, silently worrying about who had been talking, what they had been saying, and about whom.

"They are feudal in Poland!" said a loud male voice with a British accent behind my back on my second day at the Edgware Road office. I remembered the Queen of Spades saying there were some other Polish people in the office, but I never heard any reply to his remark, disappointingly. I suddenly felt as if I had gone back to school, to my former teaching job, and was being confronted by a challenging though bright pupil. The man was cheeky, but at least he knew historic words, and I felt drawn toward the owner of that voice. I turned around and there he was, the King of Clubs. A white man with short brown hair was looking at me silently from the middle of the open plan office. I was hoping it had been him speaking, and I was hoping he would continue so I could know for sure it was him, and I could respond. However, soon he too silently turned around to the row behind him, showing the back of his crisp white shirt to me and to his computer monitor. I later secretly called him "The English Peasant" to myself, though I hope he is keeping well.

I wholeheartedly wanted to connect, and yet, by my second shift, I still had no idea how to break the ice. I could not afford to lose that job. I wanted to be able to pay my rent. I so much wanted to work, and I yearned to be accepted. How do you make things good? I felt I could not reasonably say, "Are you talking about me, perhaps?" That would be exactly the kind of questions that I sometimes heard later from patients in psychiatric wards. "Are you talking about me?" "Ah, alright, so this is what you've been talking about. Because I thought you were talking about me." *Ideas of reference* is the professional word for that self-centred obsessive feeling. On my second day at Clever Costs, I may have been going through some ideas of reference, and I felt deeply unhappy.

***

"I had my appraisal last week," Paul had said one day. "Do you know what they told me during my appraisal?"

Appraisal was one of those fancy words for what they did in Paul's big office in London's financial sector. At Clever Costs, I doubt they ever did a single appraisal. For an office that size, our HR department, together with our senior management were being represented by this one person, one fair-haired young man casually seated at one of the open plan desks, on top of which my confidential paperwork rested.

"Married," said an anonymous male voice behind me at Clever Costs. "To some hopeless Polish man, probably!"

I had never been married to a Polish man, but I knew that my late Polish father and some of my other Polish family members were not hopeless, and my blood boiled, but on that occasion I did not even turn around.

***

On my third and final afternoon at Clever Costs, which was Friday, Nathan Meadowbank left early for his weekend. He stood there with his motorbike helmet under the sleeve of his office shirt. My heart was sinking because my favourite radio DJ was going to be away, and I would be left alone with nothing to hold on to except my intense feeling of not belonging. I was hoping I would be able to just focus on my workload without hearing about the "she".

I was not feeling well at all. I had felt almost physically sick that morning at the very thought of having to go to work. I felt genuinely hated at my new office and I wished there was someone senior in charge that I could turn to. I was on the run from my past, and I did not feel secure in my present at all. I was definitely no longer making 98% of the company's target. My performance must have got less than mediocre, and I felt I faced getting sacked from one more job.

A young black man, one who brought his rice and peas to work and who played football with Nathan and some other boys, leaned back in his seat, looking at me. He paused work and tilted his head, trying to catch my eye. I knew he meant well and that he wanted to get me talking in a sincere effort to put me at ease. He was the King of Hearts. However, I found myself frozen. I was unable to react. I was irrationally scared of how the rest of the staff would judge what I said. I gave him a brief look, but I was unable to ask him to discreetly look away.

"Where are you looking, Nick?" asked a male voice from the middle of the office, "Stop looking."

"She is a picture though," replied King of Hearts.

My English failed me there. I did not know whether a picture in English would be the silent one. I wished I could vanish and become visually transparent in that place.

"Don't, Nick," the Admin girl in a lovely black dress reacted instantly.

The Admin girl liked King of Hearts. She had been giving him bright lingering smiles.

"Just don't. She is… something else."

"She just thinks she is so important because she got a job in Edgware Road," said a young woman with her hijab wrapped around her face.

Edgware Road, built along an ancient Roman road, is not particularly famous other than for its range of Middle Eastern restaurants; however, it lies near central London.

"I find her repulsive," said one man with a strong African accent.

The open plan office of Clever Costs got dark as heavy clouds covered the sun outside. Large heavy drops of rain hit Edgware Road. My thoughts were with Nathan. Had he managed to get away from the rain on his bike? A lightning bolt struck close by, and we heard a powerful sound of thunder rolling through the open plan space.

"It's her!" shouted the Admin girl, my Ace of Clubs. "She made the storm!" The Admin girl ran a few steps away from her seat and squatted next to the African man's chair, the same man who had said he had found someone "repulsive". The Admin girl turned to the middle of the office to say, "I got a look so hard it made me feel so cold as never before!'

I stayed silent to the end of my shift, then walked stiffly up to King of Spades to say, "thank you for all your help", before silently leaving the office. I almost ran along the pavement in my state of a shock. So, I had been identified as the person who spurred the storm; the rainmaker of this one 21st century London office. "No-one in their right mind would ever believe me about how that place was", I thought. I later grew certain that due to the increasing stress in my life, I must have been hallucinating in that office. "How unbearably embarrassing," I decided, "to have broken down in the middle of a new workplace."

***

I never returned to Clever Costs. I briefly emailed Nathan Meadowbank to say I could not focus due to personal problems and therefore I was unable to continue work. I no longer wanted to work, and certainly not for Clever Costs, but I remembered their management had been away and I did not want young Nathan to be questioned after my failed hire. I spent the weekend in my bed, but it was not a usual lie down for me. I continuously felt intensely scared and deeply ashamed.

I could not rationalise my feelings, and instead I started having nightmares while I was awake. I was convinced that I heard various people running onto my street, sent by that Edgware Road office, to shout outside my house about how inadequate I was.

I felt like in a dream, but I also was consumed by fear. I was feverishly thinking about how to explain myself to the world. By the end of Saturday or early Sunday I wrote clusters of words in my notebook in an effort to argue my defence against my imaginary accusers and I placed the notebook on my windowsill to be read by whoever might be spying on me through it, perhaps via satellites. I now understand that I was hallucinating that weekend; I was going through my first ever psychotic episode.

***

The owner of Five Stars, Wasif, my previous long-term boss, visited me on Monday to ask what was going on with me. I got out of bed to open the front door, but then got back under my blanket as he took a chair and sat down a few steps away, near my kitchen sink. He asked about my health. I had to summon all my strength and courage to reply.

"I have gone mad, Wasif. I am mad."

"What do you mean you are mad?"

"They noticed," I insisted, "They said I was mad,"

"I don't understand," said Wasif. "Who are these people you are talking about? An office? You have been to an office where they said you were mad?"

He took off his glasses and wiped his face.

"Come back to work Kasia, you have only been away for a short time."

And that is how I returned to Five Stars. They made sure I saw a doctor, but they kept me working at their office. They kept me active, and I will always be grateful for that.

CHAPTER TWELVE – THE PATIENT

In late 2007 I was half feeling and half living. Getting back to normal after my psychosis was hard. In the first place, it felt horrible for me to hear a diagnosis like mine: psychosis. It was a Polish psychiatrist who first called me psychotic, and he did it during a conversation with my sister. This psychiatrist had never met me, but my sister met him in the summer of 2007 to ask for advice about how to talk to me. He told her I was dangerous to myself and to others. I may have had no history of violence, but to him, every psychotic patient was dangerous. I later told British doctors I was post-psychotic, and, as I described to them my paranoid thoughts during my episode, they all agreed with his remote diagnosis of psychosis.

I became scared of myself. For months, I felt too ashamed to look people in the eye and I constantly stared at the pavements to avoid accidentally glancing at other people's faces. I constantly and intensely cringed over myself, hating to see myself as a new mental health patient.

***

One London GP asked me in 2007 whether I had been thinking of harming any children. I already know that a doctor needs to ask a mental health patient about any homicidal or suicidal thoughts, but I also already know that they normally do not suggest any specific answers to that. However, after my first brief psychosis, one GP near Willesden Junction, London, asked me twice about my possible tendencies to specifically harm children, and this left me mortified. I became even more deeply scared of myself. I had been a teacher to nearly 1,000 young people before and I felt extremely strongly about child safety. I kept wondering just how dangerous I could potentially be, since it had been a doctor who asked those questions. This added to my obsession over children. I often stared at toddlers in the streets, feeling anxious about whether they were safe.

***

"Hey you! You should be smiling!" I heard on one cloudy, grey afternoon in North-west London as I was walking back home. There was a man sitting in his wheelchair beside the road. Perhaps because he was disabled himself, I did smile, shyly. He asked if I wanted him to accompany me along the street. I did want him to. I wanted somebody to help me feel less shy, and I surprisingly found enough courage to say yes when he asked. His name was Leigh. There was something very gentle about him, and he seemed to have some peaceful, cheerful strength. He looked like someone who had suddenly lost his legs, with a strong upper body. He was already an expert at wheelchair use, and he spun his chair wheels with his hands at a fast pace. We overtook a young boy whose mother kept on asking him to catch up and join her. The child whined and stayed behind.

"How can somebody with no legs be faster than somebody with two legs?" asked Leigh as we passed by the boy. The boy looked up and hurried to join his mum.

I instantly liked Leigh. I wanted to see him again. We stopped at the turn to my street, but he did not ask my phone number. I was not sure if he had any pockets on him, or a mobile phone in a pocket. Above anything else, I did not want him to feel uneasy about any questions of mine, so I never asked for his telephone number either. So, I continued to spend my evenings alone.

***

The mirror in Jeff's consulting room was tall and fairly wide. We stood in front of it looking each other in the eye in that mirror. Jeff repeatedly pushed my shoulder with his hand. My task was not to move away while going on staring back at the reflection of his eyes. He had invented this exercise to help with the new social anxiety I had complained about. Jeff was a psychiatrist, and I was a patient in his Harley Street clinic.

It was probably the last time I ever wore my old navy cardigan from Cracow, since I was embarrassed to see in the mirror that my cardigan kept riding up my belly showing off my knickers above the belt of my jeans. I instinctively pulled my cardigan down a few times, but I did not want to fiddle with my clothes too much in front of Jeff, so I mostly painfully let them be. Jeff was wearing a shirt with no tie and dark trousers. It was the first time I had fully noticed his physical appearance. He was tall and slim, perhaps slightly geeky, but I thought he looked nice.

Embarrassingly, it occurred to me the two of us together looked good in that mirror and that we would look good as a couple. I instantly judged my own thoughts as inappropriate; however, I now believe his exercises with that mirror may have been invented specifically to shift his patients' focus onto himself. I found out later on that Jeff had been banned from the medical profession for grooming his patients for sex. Some other women who had known him longer had fallen into his trap.

"Have you met Jeff? He is wonderful," I once heard some patients say about him in the lounge of a hospital where he had treated his patients before his Harley Street times.

"You are very popular," I had said to Jeff while taking a seat in his consulting room. "People talk about you."

"Oh, really?" he had replied, "And what do they say?"

It had struck me a psychiatrist would be interested to ask his patient this question.

"Only good things," I had assured him, nevertheless.

One day I had arrived at the hospital on the day of my planned appointment, just to be told briefly and rather coldly by the receptionist that Jeff was no longer working there. I did not know he had been suspended after a disciplinary procedure. So, I found him online and met him in London's Harley Street, home to many private health clinics.

***

I had a stepper with two stretchy bands for exercising my arms. My arms had always been thin, and I decided to sculpture them a bit now I was in my early 30s, so I bought a stepper with elastic bands. One morning after exercise I noticed some wet stains on my shirt although I could not remember going near the sink or splashing any water. I forgot about it, but the next morning the stains were bigger, and their positions over my breasts were unmistakable. I was obviously lactating, especially when my chest muscles worked, a side effect of a strong sedative I had been given by a Polish doctor.

Lactating only added to my distress as I sank further and further into a painful obsession over having no children. I quickly gave up exercise, although my angst lingered on. Fortunately, I did not have to complain about my side effects to Jeff. Upon his first sight of my motionless face, he wrote down in my medical records, "The patient feels insecure, not least because she is sedated." He instantly cut my dose in half. In spite of everything, I will always be grateful to Jeff for that.

I later read in a newspaper that "predator" Jeff had "showered his patients with compliments." He did. He told me I was very intelligent, and I silently craved to hear more of that. Like a good salesman, he could certainly deliver all the reassurance you wanted.

I told him about the hostile emails about me coming to

my workplace, and about the fact I found myself scared and suspicious about who else was in receipt of those emails. I wondered if the passengers on my underground platform knew about me, and then there was the laughing youth and the neighbours outside my window. Jeff would very calmly reply, "That is a normal reaction. I would have doubts too." When I complained of my inability to focus enough to read a book, although reading had been a source of great pleasure to me before, he assured me I only had to give myself some time for recovery.

"Your brain has been through an extremely difficult period and now it needs time to start functioning in the same way as before. It is as if you were complaining that, having undergone an operation on your inner organs, you were unable to run straightaway. Sooner or later, things will get back to normal."

I felt sane in Jeff's consulting room. He suggested my psychosis may have been "reactive", caused by stress "rather than a chemical imbalance" in my brain. On that basis, he said there was a chance I could recover. Because he was later banned from the medical profession, I am not certain how reliable his opinions were. Nevertheless, I was only too eager to listen. Jeff also said that my recovery would only be possible through my own hard work, and that he could only help me with some guidance. I was keen to work on my health. I was going to be the fighter with Jeff for my coach.

***

Just like Wesley had once said, Jeff believed I should learn to relax. Having listened to my concerns, especially to what I thought other people could have thought, he told me to repeat some extremely important words after him, and then to repeat them again, and again. I had paid £300 for that consultation and yet I am revealing these words to you for free. The magic words were, "So what?"

"It is not so simple though..." I interrupted.

"Repeat after me," he insisted, "So what."

"So what."

Jeff liked to quote ancient philosophers. I remember him saying you only have four basic needs in your life: air, water, nutrition, and shelter from weather extremes. So, if you worry about anything beyond those, like whether you succeed, or whether you are popular, then you should stop worrying. Keep your distance from things. Go back to the basics; that is all.

***

I also had a few appointments with a psychotherapist in Kings Cross, central London.

"Why don't we put aside your psychosis for a while and talk about your relationships instead?" she suggested. "I have noticed you have never really had a committed relationship. Before meeting your husband, you dated some men, but never for long. Therefore, is nobody good enough, or are you not good enough? Which one is it?"

"What an interesting question!" a younger cousin later said to me, "Perhaps I should also go to a psychotherapist one day if that is what it looks like. My relationships never last long, either. 'Is nobody good enough or am I not good enough', I have never thought about it before!"

CHAPTER THIRTEEN – THE DIVORCÉE

I was already in mental health treatment when I went through denial of my Clever Costs experiences. I told my psychiatrists what I believed was true, that I had first hallucinated in my new office. To be honest, my Edgware Road memories were the most difficult for me to deal with because, as time went by and as I was slowly healing from my 2007 brief psychotic episode, I was able to get control over all my other delusions and hallucinations, just not the Edgware Road ones.

In other words, I was able to slowly tell what had happened in my reality as opposed to my delusions during my psychosis. For example, I knew that in reality I had lain on my bed, while my hallucinations or delusions had been about hearing different scary people running onto my street to scream about me outside my house. I also knew that I had written different messages and drawn pictures in my notebook and that I had placed those flat onto my windowsill to try to defend my case before some imaginary invisible people in the air: I knew I had displayed my notes for real, and I knew that those judgemental invisible people floating in the air had been my delusions.

It did not feel good to know I had been psychotic; nobody wants to be ill. However, it was comforting to know that I was getting back to normal as I could tell my reality from what I had only imagined. The Edgware Road office was a hurtful black hole in my memories though, because I assumed that I had already started hallucinating in there, however there were no other memories coming back. Nothing realistic was coming back to me. I did not know what had really happened and it made me feel insecure. Everything about Clever Costs seemed to have been either a delusion or a hallucination. Had I not received my P45 paper from them, I could have believed that I had never been there at all. But, my end-of-employment paperwork arrived in the post, and I knew I truly had worked for Clever Costs for a short while. I decided to wait till my memories of that place healed and come back undistorted.

***

Encouraged by various newspaper stories of online harassers getting in trouble with the police, I decided to report Eddie's emails and phone calls. Since the disturbing emails usually arrived in other people's inboxes at my workplace, I was unable to print their contents out myself. Kama had moved back to Poland, so I could not ask her for help. I chose to approach one Ukrainian girl in our Five Stars office.

"Tanya, can I ask if you still have those emails about me in your inbox? Wasif has told me about them. I am asking because I would like to print them out for the police as evidence."

"Let me have a look. I kept deleting them, but they may still be there in my 'deleted' box."

Fortunately, the emails were still there. Tanya sent them all to print and I ended up with a hefty pile of papers. I went to my local police station in Fortune Green.

Two volunteers greeted me there. They were elderly ladies with neat short curly grey hair and lovely makeup. They decided my printouts were "not a police matter".

"You are receiving what is called spam, my dear, I receive it all the time," said one of the ladies.

"It is not spam, because it is targeted at me with my name on it. Please look at this."

I was not giving in. I was determined to stay at the police

station for as long as it took. Eventually, they stopped trying to turn me away.

"I still think it's spam, but then there is so much of it, and for the sheer volume of this pile, we will take it for the officers to see."

The other lady nodded in agreement.

"Yes, it is a police matter," said a detective to me on the phone. "Ah, our volunteers… if they thought it wasn't, why did they take it on? Anyway, we are on it. Do you know already who could be sending these to your workplace?"

"There seem to be more email addresses, and I think there may be a few people involved, with different dialects, but I believe my estranged husband would be one of them. He is away from the UK."

"Because it is an international case, it may be difficult. Don't worry, we will still deal with it, although it may take longer. First, if you have your husband's phone number, I can give him a call and there is a chance this may stop after my warning. We have classed your case as domestic harassment. I know it is happening outside your home, but, because it is by somebody from your family, we have to class it as domestic."

The detective phoned Eddie, and the emails and phone calls suddenly stopped. I was amazed, because I had suspected Eddie had been having some psychiatric problems and that he may have been unable to control his behaviour. Astonishingly though, the vision of a criminal record interrupting his career must have sobered him instantly.

***

I was thunderstruck in late 2007 when I saw an email from Clever Costs in my Customer Services inbox at Five Stars. The email came from their general address; so it would have been the Admin girl writing. My Ace of Clubs was a polished writer. Her style was impeccable as she demanded that some offensive communications to their company email must stop.

I noticed from the email thread she had copied below that they had been added to my harasser's e-mail list, and yes, those emails had been disturbing. They were mostly about my sexuality and promiscuousness, from Eddie's group of emails, as well as insults hurled back at the initial senders from Paul's email address in the thread underneath. I wrote back to Clever Costs to explain to them that Five Stars was also recipient of those offensive communications. I also explained on a more personal note that Clever Costs had received those emails because they had employed me in July. I added that my current and former colleagues, my former pupils, and my family and friends were all in receipt of the same communications, and that I had already reported this fact to the police.

The Ace of Clubs sent a neat professional email again. If she still works in administration, she must be the head of her department these days. Her second email carried three key messages, including words like: "Thank you for your reply," "'We did not know you had such problems," and "We wish you all the best." This email felt soothing to me. "We did not know you had such problems" was my favourite enclosed message, because the sentence made me feel as if they remembered who I was, but they had not known about my private problems. This made me shyly hope that I had not made any scenes during my time in their office I did not dare remember.

If my Edgware Road memories were now correct, I would still have to forgive my Ace of Clubs. I felt her second email conveyed the maximum warmth that could be enclosed in a formal style brief email on behalf of a company to one virtually unknown individual outside their business network. I was grateful for that.

***

I filed for divorce on the grounds of my husband's unreasonable behaviour. As an example of unreasonable behaviour, I briefly described Eddie harassing my work colleagues.

"Did you telephone and email the claimant's colleagues?" asked the judge.

"Yes, I did," replied Eddie, "but I am trying to explain it was not unreasonable. I would like to submit some of her emails that I have printed from her online account," Eddie took out a large pile of some printouts he had brought to the courtroom and walked over to the judge's desk. That was after I had lost access to my old email account. Eddie clearly had his access to it. The judge briefly looked at the printouts but dismissed them as irrelevant to our case.

"You have not even read all this," argued Eddie.

"I have the ability to acquire information very quickly," snapped the judge, but he added: "This has not been presented in line with the relevant procedures."

"You are siding with her because I'm black! She and I look very different, don't we!" replied Eddie.

The judge was Jewish, my lawyer had told me, and she had also said he was generally sympathetic to cases like mine.

"You have talked for most of this hearing," said the judge to Eddie. "We heard very little from the claimant, and we heard virtually nothing from Miss Day," the judge nodded at my lawyer. Eddie had arrived without a lawyer.

"I understand there is no financial claim being made. Is that right?" the judge asked, looking at me.

"That's right," I said.

Eddie was a much higher earner than me, but I considered it irrelevant to our case.

"We stopped denying women divorce 200 years ago," said the judge turning some papers on his desk.

Eddie shouted that the judge was racist, and that Eddie would file a formal complaint over the way our divorce hearing had been conducted. My first reaction was fear I might never be divorced. So, I was relieved to see the judge did not seem to be afraid.

"We can go now," whispered Miss Day to me, while I was still listening to Eddie.

She swiftly saw me out of the room while Eddie was arguing from his seat. Having asked outside if I was all right going back home on my own, Miss Day returned to the court building.

***

Klaudia finally met the man of her dreams. She moved in together with her new boyfriend of one month. I was invited to a barbecue in the house where they were renting a room together. All the other rooms were occupied by his colleagues. During the barbecue, Klaudia's white South African boyfriend gave us his opinion on black South Africans.

"I have nothing against blacks in general," Frank said, "There is nothing wrong with Wesley from your work, for example. There is nothing wrong with many blacks. It is only black South Africans that I know are stupid. We once treated our black servant to some coffee, and after she finished her coffee, she ate her Styrofoam cup. Just how stupid is that?"

Frank was the son of a wealthy man, Klaudia said; she added that his family ate with silver cutlery at his home. He must have believed he would always have an easy life even without training for a job, because he had not gone to any university, nor had he learnt any trade. He therefore worked as a cleaner in London in the noughties. On the other hand, Eddie was born into a poor shack. Eddie's lessons were often held outdoors under a tree, which was particularly inconvenient during the rain. He and his sisters often spent their lunchtime away from their classmates, hidden in their family shack, because they did not want to be seen by other children with no food for lunch.

However, Eddie was extremely studious, and he received a university scholarship after school. He was lucky to see the apartheid regime fall soon enough in his teenage years so that he could benefit from this. While a London cleaner, Frank was telling us how stupid black South Africans were, professional Eddie was working for a large American corporation. Yet, because Eddie had been harassing my colleagues, including Klaudia, I did not feel I was in a position to argue. I was generally shaky after my breakdown, so I just sat there feeling ashamed, and I did not reply.

CHAPTER FOURTEEN – THE INFORMANT

I posted an online ad on a Polish-speaking UK website in 2008. I felt lonely. Kama had moved abroad. Klaudia had cut all contact with me after she had settled down with Frank. I wanted some new friends to go out with, and a Polish community website seemed a potentially abundant source of similarly lonely, misplaced people who also wanted a new network of London friends. Indeed, I met several girls my age through that website. We were all in our 30s, all of us with no kids, all of us working and able to speak English. I was happy to have my new bunch of girlfriends.

There was chatty Bianka, elegant Beata, and straight-talking Berenika. Both Bianka and Beata lived with their English-speaking partners. I was the single one, and already a proper divorcée at the time. Bianka's husband was black, and she told us one day over lunch how annoyed she was by some other Polish girls asking her whether black men were as well-endowed as people say.

"And?" asked Beata, whose boyfriend was white, "Are they?"

We were seated in a Mediterranean restaurant, where our salads were bursting with flavour.

"And how can I know how he compares, if he has been my only man ever?" replied Bianka, a devout Catholic, who liked to make her religious ways known.

"You can't really say," I replied, "Men are not all identical. Black men vary between them just like the white men do, just like everybody has a different face. Although apparently, they sell different sizes of condoms in different countries, and I guess African men are larger on average."

"Shush, can you see this table on my left?" whispered Beata, "I think this girl has been translating our conversation to English for her friends."

A few dark-haired men and one blonde woman were seated at a table near us. Those men all turned to us, giving me smiles as I looked in their direction. Beata and I reached for our purses to pay for our meal. Bianka did not mind staying, however she joined us on our way out.

"We have to be more careful with what we talk about in restaurants," Beata said.

"Or we should go to louder places with some music on," I said.

Bianka told us she had let her spare bedroom to a fellow devout Catholic Polish woman, who later stopped paying her rent.

"I thought she had no money, and I even wanted to help her," said Bianka. "I was so angry when I found out she had been sending all her money to a monastery while paying no rent to me."

Beata had a doctor in her family, and she was our expert at all things medical. I had a spell of arthritis in my ankles in October 2008. My ankles were red, swollen, and painful enough to leave me struggling with all sorts of movement. I did walk, but I did so extremely slowly. I had the most difficulty going downstairs. My commute became slow and problematic.

Beata doubted my diagnosis. "This is not arthritis. If you had arthritis, you would feel extreme pain."

"Beata, I do feel pain though," I protested.

"No," she said, "The pain would be extreme."

Berenika was a divorced 38-year-old, who saw the rest of us less regularly. She planned to have a child or children before turning 40. She also wanted to re-marry before having a child, although she did not have a committed partner at the time. She had recently started dating an English man, but he was less perfect than her dreams. She sometimes complained to us about his poor teeth or bad looks, or she wondered aloud how much mortgage he still had to pay. She must have asked him directly, as he suddenly stopped seeing her without explanation.

***

There was a Chinese buffet near Kilburn station, in the high street. I liked their seaweed, among other dishes that I had there with a Polish man, Bartek, who I had met through the same ad as the girls, my friends-only ad. Bartek serviced the kitchen equipment in London's restaurants for a living, and he claimed never to have seen a restaurant without cockroaches in the nooks and crannies of their equipment. Taking photos was his hobby outside his day job. Bartek said he had helped his housemate with a great photo for the housemate's dating profile, which had been a success as the housemate started dating very soon afterwards, although he had ended up with a sexually transmitted disease. Bartek offered to take some high-quality photos of me with his professional camera. I decided to try that later on.

***

I changed my London address again, twice. In fact, I had read some online advice from a mental health charity that it was good to change your whereabouts after a mental health breakdown. I therefore left my Harlesden bedsit. One day in 2008, my new landlord in Camden borough asked me why I was divorced.

"Well, my ex-husband and I probably hadn't got to know each other well enough by the time we got married," I replied evasively.

My new landlord was a traditional Jew, wearing his black attire complete with a black hat over his peyote.

"I hadn't known my wife at all until our wedding day," he said. "In fact, I am not sure if I know her now. Sometimes it is better not to know your spouse too well. Well, you do have to get to know them a bit, but... the less the better, I would say."

***

I once lived in a building that was home to a brothel, the police told me. The brothel building was a multiple occupancy one where we shared our bathrooms. I never would have guessed on my own that something untoward was going on. Somebody's doorbell did keep on ringing, but I naively admired their busy social lives. I contacted the local police on an entirely unrelated matter, and I was shocked to hear about my neighbours.

"It can't be. Are you sure?" I asked the detective.

"I am positive. They leave their phone number in the local phone booths. When our officers phoned that number, the lady on the phone gave them your house address."

The detective asked me to observe the brothel to see who controlled their finances, and to speak to nobody about our conversation. He even told me later over the phone what date they were planning to raid my address. I wished I had not known. I was already post-psychotic at the time, slowly trying to reduce my medication with my doctor, and I did not feel good about the additional stress of having to be an informant. I moved out of the building soon after the police raid.

I also had a landlady in whose home – being her only tenant – I had no key to my room and my jewellery vanished.

It is tough to find the right place to live in a city like London.

CHAPTER FIFTEEN – THE PARANOIAC

In January 2009, I relapsed. I had been off medication for a while, but one day as I walked through Harlesden, I started feeling as if some people were recognising me in the street. I thought I had heard someone mention my 2007 struggles at the office that I was supposed to only have imagined. I felt scared. I phoned Jeff's secretary, but there was no reply. I went to work the next morning as usual. Somebody asked me in our office's kitchen if I was all right.

"Actually, I think I am having a relapse," I said. I thought all my colleagues knew I was post-psychotic.

"Excuse me? What are you having?"

"Ah no, nothing important."

I genuinely did not know where to seek help. Things progressed fast for me; within a couple of days I feared that somebody was perhaps using my eyes to remotely read Five Stars' paperwork, and that those mysterious people were planning to use all that random information against the laundry, to deprive me of my bastion, my workplace. I skipped days at work and this time, I received a letter of dismissal. I no longer wanted to work anyway. I became a full-time mental health patient, and I allowed myself to do all kinds of bizarre things. I guess I needed that break in my employment though.

In 2009 I started cracking down and tidying up all my memories, including those from Edgware Road. I bought some pencils and crayons and large notebooks, and I got down to drawing my Edgware Road colleagues at their desks as I remembered them. Of course, those were simple drawings, I drew stickmen, but I tried to make some of the stickmen unique, to represent the people I specifically remembered. Nathan's smiling stickman had short straight hair drawn by a carbon pencil, with a splash of yellow crayon over those carbon pencil lines. Nick's smiling stickman was wearing a bright sports top for playing football. I felt I was recalling more and more details, and I realised lots of my suspected hallucinations may have happened for real. I was beginning to nail my naughty group down; they had been real.

***

I sent a postcard to Clever Costs office in 2009. I believe it would have been a bland one, some greetings perhaps. They must have guessed I had lost it, or why would I be obsessing, so maybe they guessed I had gone properly mad. It was not just about my poor mental health that I had sent a postcard though. Sending some unexpected postcards was something I had notoriously done in my younger days to various people I had met on my way. Nowadays I try to keep in touch online with people I have liked, but in 1990s, I wrote letters to different people I could not forget. Those people often wrote back, too.

I have this very vivid good memory from my first year at college in Poland, which was before my teaching job. I was on a train to visit my parents for the weekend, and it was late autumn or early winter of 1993. That was a long-distance type of carriage with a lot of closed eight-seater compartments and a long narrow corridor on one side. I normally would have looked for a seat in one of those compartments, but the corridor was completely empty, and I chose to sit down on a small folding seat along the corridor instead. One young man in Polish military uniform went out of his compartment and he turned to me saying it was hot. Indeed, due to cold weather the heating was on, and they may have turned it up a bit too much. The young soldier kept on talking and he sat down next to me, so I must have been chatting, too.

"Really hot in here," he said again, "I cannot bear my compartment. I am expected to be wearing my undershirt, we are not allowed to take those off, as you cannot wear an incomplete uniform. We wear undershirts like this," he said, and he pulled the collar of his shirt.

He leaned toward me a bit so I could have a peek under his shirt, and I eagerly did – it was exciting to see the underlayer of a military uniform. His undershirt was crisp, it would have been ironed before he put it on. It was greenish with a crew neck, and it looked durable and thick, very practical for winter uniform.

I said it looked warm indeed. He was not even being flirtatious in any way; we were both 20 and he was behaving as if he had met his good chum and was showing off his uniform. In fact, it felt a bit like we were five. We talked and talked until the train stopped in my hometown; we were probably still talking as I got off, because I remember myself standing on the platform facing the train as he was crouching in the open door. It was a high-level floor train with steps stretching down from the doors, so he was crouching down to keep his head on the same level as my head while we were talking. I got this feeling I did not want him to disappear from my life just yet.

"Tell me your address, I'll send you a postcard," I said spontaneously.

"I should have done that, I should have given you my details, but I have nothing to write with, I can't" he said.

"Just tell me quickly and I will try to remember," I insisted. "Just say it."

He told me the address to his barracks and his full name, I repeated it with him twice, and then his train left. I kept on repeating his details to myself until I found a pen in my rucksack, and I wrote it down. Fortunately, I made it. My card must have reached him, as he sent me a letter back. He said they had made him earn my card at the barracks.

"They could see it was from a girl, so they made me do my press-ups before they gave me your card, but it was worth it. How did you remember my address?" he wrote.

His letters were always full of humour and captivating observations. He had a flair for writing; he should be writing his own memoirs now. It went on for several months, and I remember his letter that arrived in March. He was sending to me and to the other two girls in my college hotel room his best wishes on International Women's Day.

"I am sending you girls a bunch of imaginary flowers", he wrote.

I read his words aloud to the other two girls and they asked me to make sure I said thanks to him for them both.

"The girls loved your imaginary flowers," I wrote back, "We all thought they were very pretty."

***

Bianka and Beata visited me in Harlesden one day in early 2009, during my relapse after I stopped working. That was around the time I feared somebody was remotely using my eyes to spy on things. I was writing erratic messages, and I must have sent bizarre messages to Beata and Bianka. They called for the police to have me sectioned. I understood when the girls told me I had to be taken to hospital. I started packing. I packed some clothes, then some toiletries, and I also reached for a pair of small, rounded school-type scissors. Beata dashed toward me telling me to leave the scissors, so I did. I never thought much about it until I was questioned over this incident at the hospital.

"Tell me about your scissors," a doctor said to me.

"What scissors?" I asked, then I remembered. "I wanted to pack my scissors with me, and they told me to leave them."

"Why was your friend concerned over your scissors?" she continued.

"How can I know why?"

I was bitterly resentful towards Beata after getting back

home, as I realised the police had taken all my knives, even my rather blunt dinner knives from my cutlery set that I used for spreading my butter on my bread. The situation was very inconvenient for me because I had very little money and yet I had to buy some new knives to cut my food at home. I was angry. I wished I could be given at least my dining cutlery back.

"Yours is a very difficult case, and we cannot even speak to your family in Poland, because all your family have mental health problems," said a male doctor in hospital to me.

"But they don't all have mental health problems."

"Your papers say they do. Your sister has bipolar disorder…"

"My sister has no bipolar disorder. Why do you say that?"

"If it is written here that she does, then she does," was his harsh reply.

I phoned my sister.

"Have you been diagnosed with bipolar disorder" I asked.

"No. Why?"

"My psychiatrist in London thinks you are."

I then remembered the evening I had been sectioned with Beata and Bianka there with me. A blonde medic with a heavy foreign accent had talked to me at the hospital's Accident and Emergency unit that evening. She had asked me about any diagnoses I had had.

"I was diagnosed with a brief psychotic episode before," I said.

"What were you diagnosed with?" she asked.

I was visibly shaking. There was a reason I was in hospital; my anxiety was spinning out of control.

"Brief psychotic episode."

"What psychotic episode?"

"Brief. I will spell it for you if you write it down. B-R-I-E-F."

The woman started writing, but then she stopped unsure.

"Brief! Not long! Brief!" I shouted out those words.

"Ah, you mean short!" the blonde smiled broadly. "I will write, 'short psychotic episode'."

I appreciate that different foreign people, including myself, may not know all the vocabulary in English, but the woman in hospital could not understand part of my diagnosis and I hated it.

"Take her away from me!" I screamed toward the door, "She cannot speak English!"

The woman left the room and spoke to Beata and Bianka outside instead.

"Kasia, has your sister been diagnosed with normal depression or bipolar depression?" the girls came to my room to ask me. My sister had just started her short stint on anti-depressants, but I never explained it to Bianka and Beata in the hospital and I only shouted at them. This is how, to my knowledge, my sister was described in my papers as bi-polar and my whole family as mental health patients. My new acquaintances had provided all the information.

***

The police visited me again. Somebody had phoned them to say I had been trying to jump out of my window. I argued my windows did not fully open and that I only lived on the first floor, but the officers explained they had to take me to the hospital for a talk.

I was petrified that the rest of my life would look like this, with anybody else allowed to say whatever they wanted about me, and with me never getting believed. I again resented the scissors. I thought of how to badmouth people back, and I vengefully posted a photo of Beata with a male friend on my Facebook profile with an intentionally idiotic short caption, 'sex in restorant'. Bianka and Beata arrived with the police again, with Beata shouting I should be arrested. However, no doctor questioned me over Beata's concerns ever again. That was the last time I saw Beata. Bianka keeps loosely in touch on Facebook with me to this day, although she warily avoids me offline. Perhaps she stays connected online to know if I have gone mad again. Otherwise, only my older, stronger friendships survived my illness.

***

Bartek offered to give me a free photo shoot in spring 2009. It was a great distraction from my daily lack of routine. I even washed my hair for the occasion, never mind that my hair roots were of a different colour and my hair was brittle. I enjoyed posing in Regent's Park, surrounded by the greenery I had always loved. What now strikes me most in those photos is that I do not really look crazy in them. The photos show a long-haired smiling woman in her 30s, wearing a pretty net vest over her tight cotton top, and some blue beads for a bracelet. Nothing gives away either the fact that I had mostly been wearing my jogging suit, if not my pyjamas, or how deeply unhappy I was that year.

Berenika may have seen the rest of us infrequently, but when I got sectioned in 2009, she very kindly brought to my ward a few useful items she had bought, including a writing pad that I gave to a deaf fellow patient.

***

My college town in Poland had a regional centre for the deaf and dumb. There was a specialist residential school for children at the centre. They also held periodic events for deaf-and-dumb adults, who sometimes stayed over a few days in the same building where I lived as a college student. The deaf residents were known to play music extremely loudly during their stays. Perhaps some of them had some partial hearing.

The building was not a fancy one, perhaps rough for 1990s Poland. All bathrooms were shared and there was little privacy. While some big city students from dozens of miles away enjoyed living in separate little bedsits with their own bathrooms, our building only had two communal shower rooms, one for the girls and one for the boys; the communal washrooms had rows of basins for girls and boys together, and there were communal toilets with rows of cubicles for girls and boys together.

The communal shower rooms had no partitions so you could see everyone nude. I knew what bodies the other students had. Some girls felt more confident, and they casually took relaxed poses during their showers, facing the room. I was shy about my body in public, but all I could do was try and forget I was visible. I normally faced the wall.

One morning I was brushing my teeth in the communal washroom over a basin when I noticed from the corner of my eye somebody standing nearby motionless. It was a Saturday morning, when most regular students were away in their hometowns, and during that particular weekend the building had a lot of deaf-and-dumb guests. I thought the motionless person might have some mental health problems and perhaps this was why he was stood there watching. I pretended I did not notice him, trying to be polite. When I moved away from my sink though, he stepped forward and, looking at me, he moved his open hand in front of his face twice. His other hand held a razor, and in a split second I understood he was asking about mirrors. There were no mirrors in our communal washroom, so I gestured at him to come with me, and I gave him my own small mirror from my room. He soon knocked on my door to return my mirror, and I proudly felt we had had a success. We had managed to communicate. I believe people who cannot speak can be admirably creative in their non-verbal communication. All you need to do is want to understand.

***

The deaf patient seemed stranded among us hearing psychiatric patients without a sign language interpreter, and it took some time before he was transferred to a specialist unit. That is why I wanted a notepad for him, and we wrote in it together. The young man, let me call him Mike, seemed to struggle at times. He was impatient when the nurses had us play talking quiz games he could not understand. Some nurses told him off for walking around and interrupting the game.

Fortunately, one young male nurse took Mike outdoors to play basketball together a couple of times. I believe it was the nurse himself who took that initiative, so well done him.

Mike was a great dancer. He liked to watch musical shows on TV and synchronise his movements to the performers he could see. He also got me to dance salsa with him. One afternoon we danced in our day room. I made my steps to the rhythm of Mike's body movements rather than to the music I could hear.

"Let's vote for the best dancers of the ward," said one lady patient. That is how Mike and I were voted the best dancing couple of our psychiatric ward.

***

In 2009, I spent several days at one psychiatric ward at Central Middlesex Hospital. I was discharged quickly from there, even though I asked to be allowed a longer time on the ward. One lady doctor told me, "You see the hospital as your crutch, and you are trying to walk with your crutch. You do not need it. You have to walk on your own." Perhaps this was because, whenever I was surrounded by the safety of a hospital, I did well. It was only my severe anxiety that ever caused my overall mental state to deteriorate, and, in hospitals, my anxiety vanished.

During one brief hospitalisation in or around 2009, perhaps because I had no family to visit, I went to Tricycle Theatre in Kilburn for my weekend leave. They were performing "Damascus", which was about a Scottish writer of English language handbooks who visits Syria. I loved the performance.

Suddenly, the actor who played the main character forgot

his lines. The theatre went silent. I was convinced it was my personal fault. My intense attention must have caused him harm, I feared. Everything would have been my fault to me those days.

So I sat motionless, trying to shift my focus on to something else rather than him. I was clearly delusional as I believed I had interfered with his thought process. I truly was going through a relapse. However, all the hospital staff saw and knew was that I had been to a theatre while on hospital leave. I did not trust my doctor, the same one who insisted my whole family had mental illness diagnoses, enough to confide in him. I was discharged shortly afterward.

There may have also been another reason for my quick discharge. When I first got taken to hospital, and I was sectioned for 28 days that time, a Patients' Advocate visited me on the ward.

"Do you know you do not have to take medication if this is against your will?" the Patients' Advocate asked me.

I had not known that I had the choice of refusing medication. I was also startled that somebody had sent me this "messenger" to protect me from unnecessary medication. "My supporters are everywhere," I concluded with my ill mind. I told my doctors I refused to take medication. Unfortunately, the Patients' Advocate had not told me I would not be admitted to talking therapies if I were not medicated. I then never had the option of being looked after for long.

It was only after a whole year of paranoia that I went to my local mental health centre asking for medication. I swallowed my anti-psychotic tablet, and I felt instantly protected from my demons. Then I had to go to the mental health centre again, after a day or two.

"How are you feeling?" asked a passing doctor.

"I feel so much better," I assured her, "these tablets are fantastic. I feel much calmer now."

The doctor looked at me sceptically.

"Do you know that no medication works this fast?" she asked before disappearing from the corridor.

I wish I could write on social work with mental health patients. Unfortunately, I do not know anything about it. I have never had a dedicated social worker and even getting food for myself was a struggle during my relapse. Holding on to benefits had proven extremely difficult for someone with my condition living on her own.

I applied for Employment and Support Allowance in 2009, and admittedly I lived off it until my formal specialist assessment. The assessment was a profound experience for me. It was booked a long way off in London, and I worried whether I would be able to get there for the correct date and time. I tried to travel a few days earlier for some practice of moving around, but the streets looked scary to me.

Besides, I felt anxious for the birds above who I thought were suffering from dizziness. The birds definitely looked unwell to me, and I suspected even the trajectories of their flights were being influenced by some wireless waves. Somebody was controlling the birds with technology, I decided. I thought I was able to detect fragments of internet messages in the air with the power of my mind, and I particularly felt Twitter was making the birds ill in a similar way to me. I was under the impression that the birds' cries were more and more distorted till they resembled human speech. I stopped in the street clutching at my chest.

"Are you alright?" asked two policemen walking past.

I said I needed an ambulance quickly.

"It will pass. You are having a panic attack; you don't need an ambulance," replied one of the constables.

"How do you know?" I shouted angrily, which must have made them positive I did not need an ambulance at all. I was shaking agitatedly, and I remember screaming at the policemen that nobody respected them. No, my attempts to travel around prior to my ESA assessment were not a success.

I got a letter, which said my failure to attend my scheduled appointment would result in my loss of my allowance. I had no savings. I knew I had to make it to my appointment. On the big day, I summoned all my strength and despite the streets and people around me looking bizarre and distorted to me, I focused solely on the destination of my journey. Miraculously, I found the building.

There was a sign in the corridor which said "elevator". They had taught me at my English language college in Poland that "elevator" was the American counterpart for the British word, "lift". I hesitated, wondering whether I was still in the UK, but I concluded I was in London, UK, for sure. The sign on the corridor must therefore have been put up by some American intelligence agents, I speculated silently, perhaps because people's brains were so damaged.

I made it to the waiting room, and I remember speaking to the specialist assessor very briefly during my appointment. He asked whether I could travel without help. I focused to find the right answer.

"I have travelled here today on my own, therefore I can," I said.

He also asked if I could wash and dress on my own. I may have neglected myself, but I clearly recalled myself washing and dressing without help. I said I could.

The specialist didn't ask me any unusual questions.

"And how long have you been able to read other people's thoughts?" one medical professional who visited me later at my home, asked me as if out of context in Harlesden. He was smiling jovially, seated at my table together with a visiting female GP. I thought it was a slightly silly question, but I politely smiled back as I honestly replied "I wish I could. I cannot read other people's thoughts. On the contrary, I am under a machine that reads my thoughts. I have already tried to officially complain about it."

We continued to smile and talk until the end of their visit.

Not at my ESA assessment though. That assessment consisted of a few questions that were probably asked in the same form to different people suffering from different conditions. Having asked about what I could do, and having heard I could do everything he had asked about; the specialist brought my assessment to an end.

Then I received a letter saying I had no medical problems whatsoever. My allowance was discontinued. I was told to look for work and the Job Centre sent me to an employability training course with all my unhealed delusions flourishing in my head. It was probably the staff at my employability training course who informed the local mental health centre I needed help, because I had those doctors visit me at home after I had made a scene at the training centre. The decision to discontinue my Employment and Support Allowance was not reversed though. I attended my local Job Centre quite regularly in an effort to earn my Jobseekers Allowance.

***

When I did stay at hospital during my period of unemployment, as we were seated in a circle, a therapist asked us patients to introduce ourselves and say what was special about us. I said, "My name is Kasia, and I compare things." Silly as it may sound, I had decided I could compare medical treatments. I have been through different kinds of treatment, in private treatment and on the NHS, in the UK and in Poland.

In Poland, they instantly decided I was a schizophrenic that was "dis-simulating" her illness. Whatever I said was considered untrue.

"The problem you have here is that they do not believe a single word you say. I was just trying to convince them that Eddie really does exist," my sister said to me as she visited me in a Polish hospital in 2007.

The difference between my UK private treatment in Harley Street, and my NHS treatment, was that Jeff expected a lot of work from me, while in the NHS treatment I was mostly expected to be medicated and to participate in group exercises. Unlike Jeff, none of my NHS doctors ever said my recovery depended largely on myself. Perhaps this was because they were not expecting from me to recover, or perhaps because they did not want to sound judgemental. Still, I remembered Jeff's words that a psychiatrist could only guide me, but it was only my own hard work on my thinking style that could make a difference.

Jeff had asked me to buy a book on Cognitive Behavioural Therapy with some exercises in it. It was my homework to order it online, and I did. I still have a copy at home. It is called *Mind Over Mood*, by Greenberger and Padesky, and it deals with different mental health problems like depression and anxiety, but also anger, and shame. I think I had problems with all of those.

I would sit at home, get a notepad, and scribble down my thoughts as guided by the book. My biggest challenge was to be honest with myself, and yet it was the only way for those exercises to work. I was living alone, and no-one could see my notes as I finally put down the sentence, "People hate me." I still remember the way every cell of mine cringed at this sentence because I did not want to admit to myself how perpetually vulnerable and ashamed I was, but it was truly the core of how I felt at the time. Putting those words together may have been one of my milestones, because the book then guided me through, evaluating my thoughts.

In many ways, I was lucky. My strong belief is that a lot of mental health patients never get back to their active lives because they no longer believe in themselves. It is incredible how low our self-esteems can fall after periods of incapacity. For me it was perhaps easier than for many others, partly because one of my psychologists had told me she too was post-psychotic, and one doctor said she had had a lawyer patient for many years who successfully pursued her career while on the same medication as me. Therefore, although yet another NHS doctor told me I would probably never be fit for work again, I always harboured some grains of hope that I might eventually bounce back.

***

I wish I had had the comfort of a long hospitalisation during my psychotic breakdown. I hear some people are hospitalised long-term. I imagine that you probably gather strength in those long-stay units and later you don't have to deal with your memories of yourself fighting your demons on your own in the streets. I fought for my health on my own the best I could, even if it was not really for the best. When I suspected some radiation was making me sick, I rearranged items in my room and spilled a liquid medication in circles over my carpet. I washed the carpet a couple of days later only, and I am not sure all the stains came out. Because I also suspected somebody upstairs had rented their bedsit solely to install a mind reading machine over my head, I checked the staircase and unfortunately cut some cables that were fixed along the steps up. Nobody ever asked me about those cables, perhaps they were no longer in use, but clearly some of my methods of trying to heal were regrettable indeed.

CHAPTER SIXTEEN – THE NUTCASE

People want to belong. They normally want to belong with other people. During my relapse in 2009, after I stopped working, I obsessively wanted to belong with nature, and with the soil I was on. I felt as if there was a secret, but abundant source of healthy energy within the earth below my feet. Far below my feet, that is, somewhere below the layers of pavement so my feet did not reach it. In 2009, I started longing for the vast green lands I remembered from my young days in Poland. I wished I could spend my days lost between trees and clouds with nothing but mountains on the horizon. Nature can revive you, and I wanted to breathe in the pure smell of the earth. I missed having a garden outside my home, too.

***

They used a scythe to mow the grass around my grandparents' house at the turn of 1980s. A wooden pole with a wooden handlebar in the middle and a long, curved blade at the end, the scythe looked a simple tool. Using one was not simple at all; it required a lot of physical strength and some practice. They kept the pole at an angle and kind of hugged the tall grass and weeds with the sharp blade in circular, smooth, deadly strokes. The unkempt grass fell in swathes, leaving behind uneven yellowing stubs. I spent my summers there. My brother and sister, and some other children from the neighbourhood, sometimes hid in the tall grass on the days before mowing. The tall weeds along the fence always escaped the blade as the men avoided scything near hard surfaces. I could recognise some of the wild plants. There were big scary nettles that left stinging blisters on your skin, and there were bunches of fascinating touch-me-not balsam, whose ripe tiny pods full of seeds exploded at the touch of our little fingers to our amusement.

Gran sometimes dug out the pungent horseradish roots from near the fence for her kitchen, so I learnt to recognise its large leaves too. The world of plants was mostly friendly. Even the stinging nettles were said to be good for rheumatism, and we heard a story of a man who flogged his bare back with tall nettles every morning in the fields to medicate himself. The broadleaf plantain growing wild in our yard was said to have antiseptic properties; sometimes rather than ask some adults for plasters for our cuts and bruises, we wrapped our broken skins with those round plantain leaves, washed in the large tank of rainwater my grandparents kept in the yard for watering their garden. Fortunately, we never got any infections from that. Things changed over the years. As I spent my childhood summer holidays in my mum's hometown, the edge of the field behind my grandparents' house was full of wildflowers. Some other girls and I learnt to weave those flowers into little wreaths we put on our heads. The edge of the same field was full of pesticides and free from wildflowers after I grew up.

***

My first-floor bedsit in Harlesden overlooked the street. If any bedsit in our multiple-occupancy house had access to a back garden, it would not have been my little flat. The parks seemed far away to me at the time. However, the pavement outside my window had a tiny square hole carved out for a tree, and, when I felt desperately ill and unhappy, I touched the soil within that little patch with my hand. Then I sat down on that soil, pressing my back against the tree. I wanted the tree to heal me. Somebody once asked if I was alright. I said, yes, I will be alright, I just need to lean against this tree. I sometimes slept in the staircase of my house those days, curled up on the carpeted floor with my winter coat on, hiding away from my bedsit and from my huge windows overlooking the street. I was looking for peace, but there seemed to be no peace in my surroundings, and certainly there was not an ounce of peace within my anxious mind.

I had my TV and my radio in my bedsit, and I often had either one on. I saw a documentary on TV about different ethnic groups of ancient Britain. I pictured a map of Great Britain in my head with the descendants of the Celts living mostly in the north, and the descendants of the Anglo-Saxons settled predominantly in my country of residence, England. The documentary said the Celts were a stronghold of Christianity when the Anglo-Saxons tended to revert to paganism. I had been born into a Catholic family and I had never felt drawn to paganism before, but I wanted to belong with the Anglo-Saxon ashes of this soil I was on. I focused on the pictures they showed on TV. They showed a picture of an altar as they spoke about religion. There was a cross in the centre as they spoke about Christianity, and a large skull of a bull or cow as they spoke about Anglo-Saxon pagans. I wanted a skull for myself, too.

I could not think of where to find a cow's skull, but I certainly knew where to find a sheep's skull instead. There were some Muslim butchers at a supermarket nearby. I went there and asked the boys if they had any sheep's skulls in their freezer at the back. A lot of Middle Eastern and African people cook sheep skulls for a special soup; it is considered highly nutritious or a delicacy for their guests. I remembered from my own time working for a Middle Eastern deli shop that skulls would normally be kept in a freezer away from the counter. Indeed, the boys told me to wait at the counter until they brought me a skull. I took it home, but I did not cook with it. I took some photos instead. The skull still had the brain inside, but it was wrapped in a white plastic bag very tightly, so I left the bag on and put the skull on the floor. I arranged a dark green anorak as the body for this skull and I then took photos of this fantasy creature as if it was crawling upstairs or standing in my room, with my arm holding the skull, my arm fully covered with the anorak. I had my own dragon at home, perhaps one for England's patron St George to fight. I spent my night with the skull in my room, taking pictures and listening to music by Mumford & Sons as it was the only music I felt was related to English folk, and also because I truly loved their music. The skull, wrapped in layers of plastic, got dumped in the bin outside my house at dawn. I felt that I was now just like the ancient Anglo-Saxons who rested in this earth, and who seemed to me to have cherished animal skulls.

***

One day in Harlesden, when I was ill, I was standing in line for a cashpoint. I looked a mess as I hardly changed my clothes or washed or did anything with my hair those days. There were some well-groomed pretty girls in front of me who turned back to have a look at me. One of the girls perused me before whispering to the other one who also turned to look me up and down. I suddenly felt a surge of fury inside the whole of me. I stood in silence for a while, with growing anger and frustration at being stared at, and finally I stepped forward and pushed them away from the queue.

"Go away! Get away from here!" I screamed.

They had not been speaking English and, at the time, I wished them out of London altogether. I felt they were some non-empathetic invaders. Surprisingly, they quietly went away after my push. I saw the silent, uneasy looks from the other people in the queue ahead.

"I am mad!" I shouted.

Nothing happened. Then I thought perhaps I could get priority in the queue for being mad. I pushed the person in front of me and took their place, shouting I was mad. Then again, and again, until I was first in queue. When I was at the very front, I felt a push and I stepped aside. A young black man took back his correct place at the front of the queue. He was silent and he looked ahead with a blank gloomy stare. He looked unhappy to me.

"Brother," I said. And I started weeping, with tears running down my face and audible sobs breaking out of my chest. I cannot justify or explain it now, especially as I do not usually cry at all. I normally hate tears, but huge tears were rolling down my face as I used the cashpoint. I was probably crying for myself and for that "brother", and for any other potential mental health patients around. There was no bed in the nearby hospital for me at the time, the local wards were full, such was the demand for mental health care in that area. When I turned back with some cash in my hand, there was no-one left in the queue behind me. The pavement was empty.

Sometimes I tried to understand what was wrong, and why things looked strange to me; I came up with different scenarios of what had happened to the world, rather than to me. I tried to solve endless riddles, thinking there had been some magnetic field discharge that damaged people's brains. I thought something needed to be done. I bought small food items from various parts of the world and tried to write about different cultures. That was how I ended up scanning my nonsensical sentences at Ghais's internet café. I sometimes shouted from my window, too.

***

When I felt entirely disconnected from any organised life, I sought consolation in the area's history to forget the poverty of my own place in it, or the litter in the local streets that lured the city foxes.

Brent Council said on their website "Harlesden, originally 'Herewulf's Tun' ('Herewulf's Farmstead'), began as a

Saxon settlement on an elevated and well-watered woodland clearing." Having found this information online at Ghais's, I searched further to find that the Old English male name "Herewulf", in turn, combines two Old Saxon word stems: "heri" or "army", and "wulf" or "wolf".

I felt it was romantic to live on the same patch of earth where a Saxon called "Armywolf" would have settled around the 5th century. I love historic names and foreign languages. They tell me about their speakers. Words are like enthralling artefacts moulded by the strength of human thought.

We know from historic language about how special wolves were to the Saxons. Names like Herewulf or famous Beowulf, or Wulfweard, suggest human connection with the animal world. By calling their son "wolf", what qualities did they hope to be passing on to the child?

I kept on delving into the history of the area. I visited the nearby graveyard to see who had lived in the neighbourhood. There was a tombstone of a captain who had died at sea. The tombstone would have been empty, but I found it inspiring. The captain of Harlesden or of nearby Kensal, I hoped his spirit would help me navigate.

***

I sought to heal through my old friend art. I had gone to a contemporary art event in one of London's parks to see what people were creating. The exhibition was called "Frieze", and it was advertised on TV with a slogan, 'If you're not there, you're nowhere.' There were works of art from different countries. Some of the works showed less apparent skill, like a simplified human shape cut out of a piece of paper. There were also elaborate paintings, like an oil-on-canvas series depicting group sex. I must admit that this artist had talent. The naked bodies were beautifully painted with strong brush strokes, with all the subtleties of colour within the controversial theme.

As I walked on, I saw a soft toy lying on the floor, a grey

alien with large eyes and with a large red penis. Since there were young children around the installations, I personally felt uneasy, but I guess I am just old school. If I had had the money, I would have bought a huge oil painting of some turquoise water and fish in it. Then there was a set of erotic photos, and I thought to myself I could probably take better ones. And there was a large cross with a huge bright green stuffed frog on it. As I later walked through the streets wearing my bright green jogging suit, I thought to myself that I must have looked like the green frog on the cross.

There was an old satellite dish outside my window in Harlesden Gardens. I decided to turn it into my own work of art. I bought a can of mint green paint nearby and a flat medium brush. I somehow wrote "Free Intelligence" across that dish with my mint green paint. Then I dipped my brush in this paint again, let it dry, and attached the brush upright to the mast clamp with some clear tape. I loved the plucky look of the personal, modern coat of arms I had just invented and claimed. I admired my work until my landlord came with a can of black spray paint, tore the brush off the mast and covered my satellite dish with black paint, till my mint green slogan was no more.

I did my own performative street art that only I understood. My performances ranged from running around my home with various accessories to jumping and dancing to imaginary music. You would not have wanted to see me at the time. The irrational is often scary.

***

Having been repeatedly turned down by my local Accident and Emergency unit for in-patient mental health treatment, I eventually tried to fight for a hospital bed. I went to my local psychiatric unit, and as a nurse opened the door to her ward, I tried to squeeze in. I kept my foot in the doorway. The nurses phoned the police. Two officers took me out of the unit and put me at the back of their vehicle behind some bars. They asked me where to drive to, and I said somewhere I finally could sleep. Then they stopped in front of a large hotel saying I could sleep there. I sat down on the curb beside the road, but they stopped their car and came back to me. They said I could not sit on the curb and to go to the hotel instead. I finally walked into the hotel, where a sympathetic waiter gave me a free apple before the security saw me out of their door. Then I somehow managed to find my way back home.

***

As I re-lived some of my first psychotic episode's fears, I started worrying about Paul again. In the end I recalled his details and found him online to check if he was OK. Paul arrived at my new address and hugged me affectionately. Perhaps he had missed me after all. I was happy to have him around, although in the midst of my delusions, seeing him felt unreal.

"I have changed," I said quietly as were seated together, but I couldn't bring myself to tell him exactly what had been going on with me. I went silent.

"Yes, I can see," he whispered.

Paul's life had not changed much. He was still temporarily living with his parents after selling a home he had shared with his ex-wife. The main news was that he had taken up a dance course. I was vividly interested in that development, and we ended up dancing in my bedsit. He showed off some steps he had learnt. It was fun.

"I can stay with you," he looked at me. "I can sleep here. You always wanted me to stay with you overnight."

"No, you can't," I protested, "you must go now. Please just go."

He was right to believe that I wanted him to stay. Sharing our morning would have been my old dream come true. However, I thought it was too late, my life had capsized since the last time we had met. In my ill mind, I feared I was likely to die overnight, and my broken logic was that he would get imprisoned after waking up next to my cold, lifeless corpse. I felt keeping my distance was the best I could do for this man that was so dear to me. I then wrote to him that I was going away and therefore could not meet anymore.

CHAPTER SEVENTEEN – THE CONVALESCENT

I had spells of sanity in 2009. Whenever I felt better, I hungrily searched for all kinds of advice online from organisations devoted to mental health. As I said, I learnt it is good to move to a different location after your breakdown. In early 2010, I decided to finally use my strong advantage and privilege of being able to move back to my parents' old home, away from my Harlesden bedsit.

Booking a flight seemed too complicated for me at the time. Instead, I bought a coach ticket to Poland. Travel by coach was going to take at least one day and night, but it would take me directly to my home district, so it seemed an easier option. The international bus station in Victoria was packed with people. The electronic noticeboards displayed rows of destinations that kept moving up. I found it challenging to try and match the information on the display boards with the different buses approaching different gates. I got scared that I might never make the journey. Eventually, I found the correct gate, and I heard a young Polish couple talking about their coach. They were headed toward the same destination as I was. I thought holding on to them would increase my chances of catching the correct vehicle.

"Przepraszam bardzo," I said to them in Polish, "Excuse me, are you travelling by the 3 o'clock coach to Cieszyn?"

They confirmed, looking at me distrustfully.

"Please help me. I am heavily medicated, and I fear I may

miss my bus as I find it difficult to focus. Please let me know when our coach arrives, do make sure I board it with you."

They pair looked at me and at each other.

"We will let you know," the man replied.

As I later dozed off on a nearby seat, the man shook my shoulder to help me board.

My ailing mum welcomed me back at her home in Poland in 2010. Mum's home may not have been wealthy, and I was unemployed, but the home had a garden. I took my old easel and paints outdoors in the summer and I painted some garden views over my old canvas. It was a tranquil feeling. The stirred pieces of my mind took many months to fall back in place. However, having a loving family member around me had a healing effect. There was somebody near me that I cared about. I was no longer in a void. Mum was my motivation to make my daily effort and hopefully to behave in an acceptable way.

I did not want to disappoint my mum, so I put on a sane manner, which was good as I later had no fresh embarrassing memories of myself to deal with. I was also no longer hungry as my mother did most of the cooking. I felt reassuringly safe when it came to the most basic level of biological needs, and I felt someone cared about me. My slow healing process kicked in.

***

Applying for jobs was always something I planned to do again. I do not believe I was quite ready for employment in 2011, but I tried for vacancies I hoped to do well at. In Poland, there was a scheme at the time where the employment of disabled people was partially funded by the government. Some poorly paid job offers were specifically intended for those registered as disabled. I applied for my disability paperwork, and I got my psychiatric certificate. Just in case, I said at my job interviews that I had got my certificate for depression. I thought depression sounded better than psychosis. People are very tolerant of mental health patients nowadays, unless someone previously diagnosed with a severe condition wants to pursue a responsible role. It is a complex issue. They tend to explain all unacceptable behaviours by psychiatric diagnoses. I have seen a British TV documentary about a murderer who had a history of depression and anxiety, and who was diagnosed with borderline personality disorder. They said it as if this diagnosis explained the murder. I also have a history of depression and anxiety now, and I too was once diagnosed with borderline personality disorder. I received even more diagnoses, like psychotic episode, schizoaffective disorder, and schizophrenia.

Whether or not my diagnoses have all been accurate, I would rather people did not see me as a potential killer. I had heard from a couple of doctors about some other post-psychotic people continuing with their professional careers; however apparently those people had all kept their medical histories secret. My one British nurse had warned me not to disclose my medical history to potential employers, and perhaps to write in my CV instead that I had been travelling for a year. I did not lie in my CV, but I understood very clearly that I could not afford for my diagnoses to be known to my potential employer.

I was lucky. I found a rare job ad for a disabled person to help at an office in return for the Polish minimum wage. Mostly, the disability jobs were for cleaners or CCTV operators. I took my disability certificate with me to my job interview, and I was hired. My new beginnings at work were not easy for me, because I was obsessing over having a secret to hide. In all honesty, I did not do much in that job; I struggled there. Every time I heard some lowered voices, or some people giggling, I panicked they were talking about me. I imagined how angry my employer could get if they learnt I was post-psychotic and not just depressed. In my mind I went through the most embarrassing memories of my illness again and again. In the end, I did what I should have done in 2007 at Clever Costs: I took long-term sick leave.

***

In 2011, I joined an outpatient group therapy at a mental health hospital in Poland. We spent months seeing each other every morning, and I made some friends. We did assertiveness role-play exercises, and we made drawings that were later analysed in our group. The patients had different conditions, and one depressed female patient elaborated one morning about how morbid psychotic people were. Another post-psychotic patient got very upset about that. "The therapists should not have let her speak," the post-psychotic patient said to me.

One group exercise that we did was a map of our group's social dynamics. We wrote down our names on a large sheet of paper, and then we drew arrows from our names to three other people's names. Those were meant to be the people we respected or those we would like to share our experiences with. I cannot remember precisely the categories, but I remember I got the biggest number of arrows in our group. That was supposed to mean I was popular in our group. However, I do not know how this was meant to help those patients who got very few arrows.

***

I started looking for new international friends on an internet site called Badoo. Before I realised everyone else seemed to be looking there for sex, I met a French male resident of Poland, Xavier, for a drink at a pub. He was a very handsome young man in his 20s. Initially, I was tempted to forget our age difference when he mentioned romance. However, the longer I looked at him, the younger he seemed to me. I imagined his family's faces if they could see me drinking with him at that pub.

"You really are very young," I said, "and I should be going. Of course, you can talk to me anytime you want.

136

Perhaps I can give you my Facebook details so we can stay in touch."

"I don't have a Facebook profile. I use other online platforms," he said. Then he added through his teeth, "Facebook is for old people."

I smiled and nodded my head toward him. "Fair enough," I thought.

***

The Polish dating site that I subsequently joined used the traditional words for your relationship status: "kawaler" or "bachelor" and "panna" or "spinster" were options for those who had never been married. Even though my divorce had been a bad one, I was still relieved I did not have to call myself a spinster at around 40. I had uneasy memories from my youth, when an old spinster was someone that you did not want to be.

"Don't sit at the corner of the table or you may end up an old spinster," Granny would say.

Old bachelors and old spinsters of my young days were generally ill-adjusted, but the women were particularly bad, according to common knowledge.

"She is very unkind, but then what can you expect of an old spinster?" one my ex-pupils told me about my colleague.

"I know. I am an old spinster myself," I replied, partially through solidarity with the other woman, because I was only in my mid-20s at the time.

"No, you're not!" said he, "How can you even compare yourself! She is really mean!"

In your late 20s, people normally began to worry for you if you were not yet planning to marry.

"My colleagues have started banging their wedding rings against their desks at me," a single male friend told me once, "Time for me to start thinking of someone to marry."

I must admit I suspected the man of being a fantasist at first, because I had never seen anyone banging their wedding rings at anyone. However, one my female friends from college later complained of precisely the same. Her colleagues had also banged their wedding rings at her. She also soon started dating someone as she felt their pressure to do so. You had to be resilient in those days, even as late as the 1990s, to go against the flow in Poland.

As usual, I had filtered my dating site for a man with a degree, or at least with secondary education, and taller than me. I found a relatively local man who I liked. Tomek was a bachelor and a musician who played the organ during church services for a living. He preferred playing his electric guitar, but playing the organ paid his bills.

His job as a church musician seemed very symbolic of 21st century Poland. While Polish communist authorities had made it very clear you were not supposed to follow any religion, the authorities of 2010s Poland made it very clear that the Roman Catholic Church was in favour. Lots of funds went to the Polish bishops those days, and Tomek could make a living through the connection. Personally, I wish the Polish authorities would stop trying to supervise people's minds. I was no longer a regular churchgoer in the 2010s. From my younger days I remember that religious meditation can be a fabulous source of serene strength; however, I no longer seemed to derive much strength from religion. I hadn't done since my late 30s. I no longer believed in the power of my prayer, so prayer gave me no resilience anymore. God for me was this powerful natural force that instigates life, but I kept my distance from organised religion.

***

Tomek was a lovely person, but he was Polish like me, and he planned to stay in his local area of Poland for the rest of his life. I was not sure I would be happy living there forever, and we finally parted as good friends. I thought of going back to the UK. I had fallen ill in London, and my irrational but strong feeling was that I could only fully recover in London. I felt like a fugitive without trying to face my old surroundings and old ghosts again.

Besides, I struggled with my job search in our local area. I was around 40 and, in Poland, I seemed to be too old to restart my career. Polish companies were very clear that they looked for "young and adaptable" staff, especially for all junior positions. You are expected to be in your 20s in Poland's job market. Even in the UK, the Polish-speaking job boards often feature Polish companies based in Great Britain that promise to their candidates they would be working in "a young dynamic team".

"I have some administrative work experience from England, and I did a bookkeeping course in London," I said during one my job interview in 2013 Poland.

"...Which is of completely no use in Poland," replied Bogdan, the company boss.

After that interview, Bogdan himself phoned my number.

"The administrative vacancy has now been filled," he said over the phone, "but we are looking for the security control room operative for our company. Would you be interested in that?"

I ate my humble pie and accepted that job. It was not what I had wanted, but after all, I did need a job, and I could not find anything else. I was 40 in 2013 and too old for a new office job in Poland without some thorough local experience. Nobody needed a full-time English teacher nearby. I started doing my 16-hour shifts from 4pm to 8am at their control room.

***

My control room job turned out to be more responsible than I had expected. It was my responsibility to make sure all our remote staff and their locations were safe overnight. I periodically received electronic signals from their hand scanners as they patrolled their premises. Between their patrols, I phoned my remote colleagues to make sure they were safe, and unofficially, to ensure they were awake.

"Witam panie Darku, Hello mister Darek, how are things going at your end?" I said as I phoned one our security staff.

"Pani Kasiu, Ms Kasia, things are just like in a Polish movie here, completely nothing is going on. No action."

***

I kept checking London job ads and I eventually found a potential employer who phoned me back. They were looking for somebody with bookkeeping skills to work for them on the minimum wage. I moved to the UK and started working for them within a month. I felt very grateful to fate, or to my God, for being back in age-tolerant United Kingdom. I finally had my new office job again, something already unthinkable for me in Poland at the time.

My return to the UK in 2015 was different to my first steps in this country back in 2003. Probably the main difference was that a job was waiting for me, so I no longer had to go through the pain of having to find somewhere fast. That was fortunate for me, because I lacked the peaceful confidence I used to have, and therefore I could have struggled with a new job hunt.

CHAPTER EIGHTEEN – THE CONFIDANTE

"You look beautiful in your passport photo," said my new line manager in 2015 while scanning my passport for my employee file on my first day at A-to-Z Products Ltd.

"Oh, come on, I look awful," I said. My photo showed a fat face. I was no longer slim in the 2010s. Weight gain is a common side effect of the medication I was on, and I had not yet learned to manage my weight while taking my tablets.

"Why?" my new manager looked at my photo again.

I wondered how anybody could like this photo of mine, and I suddenly realised my new manager was of Indian origin, with thick black eyebrows and dark eyes. Perhaps he may have liked my complexion or my eyes. People so often like what they do not have. I personally used to admire the looks of some of the Kurdish girls at The World Food Deli in 2003.

"You are so lucky," I once said to my former manager Emir's fiancée in 2003, "You don't have to paint your eyebrows. You have perfect eyebrows and eyelashes, not like me."

"Are you serious?" she replied, "I am too hairy. Look at the dark hairs on my arms. It is you who is lucky, as your hairs hardly show at all."

"I never thought about it," I said. "It's just that my eyebrows or eyelashes don't show either. Without makeup, my face looks totally plain."

"But you must have brought your suntan from somewhere hot, Missy!" the middle-aged lifeguard shouted after me, joking about my pale skin at a swimming pool in late 1990s Poland.

In 1980s and 90s Poland, you were supposed to be suntanned, especially in the summer. During my school holidays in the 80s, at summer camps, our teachers set aside time for us teenagers to sunbathe as we lay flat in the scorching sun. We later compared our skin shades. Some kids were triumphant about their successfully brown tan. I was usually burnt red by the sun, or my skin had only a very light golden hue at best. I was always the whitest in my group.

"Your legs look very white. They don't look good. You should wear some longer clothes over them. Why don't you try to get tanned today?" my mother would say.

It was only in the UK in 2000s that I noticed some snow-white girls showing off their skins in the summer, without anyone staring or shouting at them for being too pale. It was fantastic for me to see their confidence. They made me feel less shy about my own skin shade.

***

My new manager's name was Saihaj. He was in his 20s.

"I cannot say I am like your older brother," he said to me during his first one-to-one meeting with me, "because you are the older one, but I am indeed like your brother. You can always talk to me, and you can tell me any of your problems."

I liked Saihaj. I was his first direct report ever, and I felt he was trying to make things work.

There were more Asian employees in the company.

"One thing I would like to mention is cleanliness," said our new English director, Rod, who had moved down from a town in northern England where they may have had fewer ethnic minorities. "I have had a look at different staff toilets today, and they are untidy. Also, what are all those plastic bottles lying about? Surely, after drinking your water you could put your bottle in the bin."

I was opening my mouth to explain those bottles were probably for ablutions, when a young Indian man, Pradav, spoke out.

"These are for washing your thingy after you've done your toilet. It's an Asian way."

I had not known it was an Asian way, and not only an Islamic way. Rod looked stunned, and he quickly ended this part of his speech.

"I think Rod is a little bit racist," said Pradav to Saihaj after the meeting. Then Pradav looked at me.

"Oh, don't worry about Kasia," Saihaj said quickly, "She will not say anything. I know her and she won't go and speak to Rod about it."

***

We regularly changed the door codes in our office. Saihaj showed me how to dismantle the key-in door locks, how to change the position of the tiny red plates inside to set a new code, and how to mount the locks back onto the doors. After several weeks, it was my turn to show the same to our new hire, Pradav. On the same day, I took some files back into our archive closet. I let the closet door close behind me as I rearranged the files neatly on the shelf. However, as I made my way out, the door lock refused to open.

I had checked Pradav's locks on our other doors, but I had forgotten to check the closet lock, which was rarely used. The handle inside the closet had not been attached to the lock's mechanism properly. In a way, I was relieved it was me, and not someone else, who had got stuck inside. Still, I did not know how to get out.

"Help!" I knocked on the closet door from the inside, but there was no-one there to hear me.

I looked around for a screwdriver, but there was none.

I imagined myself spending the night in the closet through the night. I had to do something. There was a clothes hanger made of a thin wire. I thought I could use the wire instead of a screwdriver, if only I found a way to flatten the ending a bit. Then I heard somebody flush the guest toilet, which was near my closet. I heard somebody step out, and I started banging on my closet door.

"What the hell?" I heard our boss's voice in the corridor.

I shouted and knocked until the door was opened from the outside and I saw his bewildered face before me.

"Thank you so much," I grinned.

Then I fetched a screwdriver to fix the lock.

***

I did tell my one UK boss that I was post-psychotic. After a year of employment, my boss asked me to attend a customer meeting in the absence of a sick colleague, but I panicked. I said there was no point of me going. I would probably have blown their meeting anyway, because I felt hysterically scared the customer could recognise me as a mad woman who used to walk the streets saying stupid things. People tend to fail when they panic, and I most certainly would have.

However, after a few more months we were short-staffed again, and I said to my boss I would be happy to go to one customer meeting. I felt ready, and I was right, as the meeting turned a success. It was an incredible boost to my confidence in the field of my work.

Being known to my colleagues for my mental health struggles produced a surprising dimension. Some colleagues seemed more comfortable telling me about their own problems. One lady phoned my private mobile number to say she had just had her first panic attack ever, and that she was planning to be absent from work for an unforeseeable time. I spoke to her line manager for her.

"And what do you think about it?" her manager asked me.

"I think she's going to be fine soon," I said, feeling like an expert in the field. "You can learn to manage these conditions and I'm sure she will. She is just panicking the first time."

"She has to get a grip of herself," her manager said, "And I know what I'm saying because I also used to have panic attacks."

On another occasion, a male colleague confided in me he was feeling anxious about things.

"Do you ever have dreams that repeat themselves?" he asked me.

I felt his question may have been important to him; I was suspecting he might be a fellow patient, so I tried to recall some dreams.

"I used to have repetitive dreams about myself falling," I replied, "I would sometimes wake up stretching my arms for protection. Then it all went away."

"What about in real life? Do you believe you can go through the same situation again and again? And if so, what would you do? If you see the same thing again and again?"

"I am not sure you can go through precisely the same thing. Something would always be different. The point of time would be different. Besides, you would be different. You would have been through different experiences. After you have dealt with a situation once, you may have developed some new coping skills that could help you deal with a similar situation later. You develop new skills as you go."

"I had never thought about that," he said, "thank you, it was helpful."

***

I once received a phone call from the male owner of a cheerful and confident voice. The man on the phone chatted for a few moments and he recognised my name as Polish.

"I am thoroughly familiar with all things Polish as I have worked with a lot of Polish customers and colleagues," he said.

His chatter put me in my relaxed mode.

"I thought you were going to say you had a Polish girlfriend, like everyone else," I said.

"No, a man of my cali…" said the cheerful and confident voice, and then he suddenly paused. It was as sharp as the cut of a knife, his silence. It was not a stutter. He just stopped talking and it occurred to me he may have suddenly realised he was talking to a Pole. "A man of my calibre does not have a Polish girlfriend," I finished his thought in my mind, but I said nothing. I did not know how to help him out. I froze as he froze, and I waited for his next word I could hold on to.

"I am too busy to have a girlfriend", he finally said in a rather dry voice, and he quickly jumped on to the business matter he had wanted to talk about. I eagerly joined him in that business talk. Only after we hung up, I put my face in my hands. "A man of my calibre," I whispered with a giggle. What an accidental comedian he had been without saying anything at all.

***

I moved from one office to another in pursuit of a higher salary. I met a wonderful colleague at one office. Her name was Shravya, and her family hailed from India. I showed Shravya around our office on her first day, and we spent her first lunch break together.

"I hope they are respectful here," she said. "I have seen bullying in some offices before. At one of my former workplaces, a colleague next to me said 'Asian women are good for breeding'."

I assured Shravya she should not worry. I had known our other colleagues long enough to be certain they would be respectful.

She was sharp as a razor, Shravya. She thought clearly and she would have not misunderstood that comment about Asian women. I suddenly realised it would have been perfectly possible for me to hear comments like "Married, to some hopeless Polish man, probably," for real, too.

***

One company, I'll call them "Expat Services", was looking for a translator. I was invited to their interview. The practical tests with them were a breeze to me. I passed their data entry test and another test advising someone over the phone in English. Then they invited me for a final chat where I briefly mentioned being on antidepressants. The two interviewers looked at each other. After the interview, I received an email saying I was being turned down for not having enough translating experience. I had chatted to some other candidates earlier, and I knew I had more translating experience than most of the candidates did. After that, I never mentioned my mental health again when trying for new jobs.

CHAPTER NINETEEN – HIGHLAND REEL

There was a minicab company at the top of my road in London in 2017. An Afghan driver picked me up one day. As with many similar drivers, he asked me if I was married and had children. I said I had a boyfriend.

"What nationality is your boyfriend?" he asked.

"Scottish."

"At least, not English," he said. "I have a lot of English customers. They usually drink beer and talk about football. And I think to myself, in the evening this man probably sits down in his bedroom with a beer in his hand and talks about football. What kind of life does one have with a man like that?"

I knew that in the UK football, just like all other kinds of sports, is considered a safe, generic topic for conversation, and I thought his customers might have simply tried to stay within some non-offensive topics for conversation. But, different people read different things into the same experiences.

***

As a mental health patient in 2009, I had been offered a kind of a course in "small talk" within my therapy group. We were advised to keep ourselves updated on sports, weather, celebrity lives and entertainment and then use that information for small talk in our group. We were warned not to talk about religion or wars.

"And what else is there to talk about?!" asked one older Pashtun patient, Irfan, in exasperation. Irfan was never able to avoid mentioning religion or war during our exercises and he was repeatedly rebuked by our therapist.

There was another cultural exercise we did. The therapist played different pop songs and asked what we had been doing on hearing them for the first time. The Britons in our group told us their stories seamlessly. They all seemed to remember every detail of their lives against the music they had heard. I struggled.

"I really don't remember when I first heard it, though of course I heard it many times," I said, "Perhaps I can say instead how the music makes me feel?"

The therapist was not impressed by my suggestion.

"I don't know this song," Irfan said.

***

As he was divorced, liked the gym, had a degree and was taller than me, Cameron instantly came up in my online dating service search in 2015, while I was preparing to move from Poland to the UK again. He was the first person in his family to earn a degree, and I now thank God he did, or I may have never found him otherwise. I loved Cameron's face in his profile photo, but I also liked his down-to-earth description of himself. I messaged him first.

He did not seem particularly interested in me, but he replied politely to all my messages. I later learned he had been going through bereavement, and he had not been actively using this dating website after signing up. He had apparently ignored some other women's "silly" messages, but he felt that I was very genuine and "even if I asked how he was, it felt like I really cared to know the answer." So, he did not want to be rude to me, and he kept on replying. From my point of view at the time, all I could see was that he was just being polite rather than very keen on dating me. However, I liked him a lot, so I chose to pursue friendship with him rather than to date anyone else from that website. And then we got on like a house on fire, spending hours on the phone at the evenings and weekends, before meeting in person when our romantic relationship started.

My extremely low self-esteem did not help me when it came to building a lasting relationship. From the start I had thoroughly enjoyed talking to Cameron, but when we first met, it was in a crowded place, and I had an anxiety attack due to being among so many people. I got better after we left the place. I generally felt best when meeting at home and I felt anxious whenever we were about to go out somewhere together.

"I am always afraid somebody could recognise me as the mad woman and say something unpleasant to you," I finally said; it took a mountain of courage for me even to say that to him.

"Don't worry about things like that," Cameron tried to convince me, though I continued to worry.

As time went by, I got to know the cheeky joker he apparently had normally always been, and he also got to see my relaxed side a lot. My healing process gathered speed as I thrived next to his confident personality and a lot of my old trauma faded. I had probably never laughed as much in my life as I did around Cameron. We did silly things when no-one was watching, for example we played this game at some point, where I ran across the room repeatedly as he tried to throw a ball of soft kitchen tissue at my moving head.

***

In early 2017 I felt ready for a new professional challenge. My CV made me look like a job hopper, and the usual response to my new job applications was rejection emails. I did not want to give up though. I posted my free jobseeker ad on Gumtree website, which was still possible at the time, where I said I had some administrative and bookkeeping experience and made "good tea". I received a response from Trevor Fairfield of an engineering company, Celestial Circuits, requesting my CV. I loved his interview.

"The job is yours," he said at the end. "We have mostly boys here. The main topics for conversation are football, cars, and women, and everyone specialises in one of these. You will fit in."

Celestial Circuits was my first office with a dress code outlined in my contract. The dress code was to be smart-casual, which was perhaps a step up from my entirely casual clothes at my earlier workplaces. So I did some shopping for clothes.

***

"It is very easy to check if your skirt is the proper length," said the female religious moderator to our group of girls at one Catholic retreat in 1990s Poland. "When you kneel, the skirt needs to touch the surface you are kneeling on. This way you know you have a modest length. Do not buy any clothes with a low-cut neck, and it is best to choose a short sleeve over any sleeveless tops."

I may have drifted away from organised religion by the 2010s, but as I tried to choose some professional tops for work in 2017, I still found myself influenced by those old rules. I despaired over how the majority of work tops in the British shops seemed to have their necks cut low. Previously, I would wear casual tops with a boat neck at best, and I had steered clear of V-shaped low necks. In 2017, I did eventually buy some blouses that showed the top of my cleavage. I simply pulled those blouses repeatedly to my back as I wore them, to minimise the amount of my body showing below my neck at the front.

***

Celestial Circuits was a lively and colourful workplace.

There were some quick-witted people, and I laughed a lot at their conversations. I could not speak in a similar way, and I felt their jokes at me were less sharp as they made allowances for my foreign kind of English. The workplace did have its problems, too. I once witnessed our office manager, Donna, clash with one project manager, Toby in the office.

"Would you describe Toby's behaviour as aggressive?" Trevor asked me in his office.

"No, I would not describe him as more aggressive than Donna was. I do not believe there was a clear victim during that incident. It was more like two strong personalities clashing."

I knew Trevor would have preferred for me to side with Donna. Donna and Trevor often held hands despite him living with his wife. Single Donna was genuinely crazy over Trevor, and she was clearly hoping he would settle down with her eventually.

They said our storeman, Tyler, had nearly lost his job after opening a parcel at work that contained some Viagra pills. Tyler had finally checked the exact address on the parcel and taken the Viagra to Trevor's office muttering, "Erm, I think this would be yours, boss."

The boys in the office disapproved of Trevor and Donna.

"Oh no, not them again!" moaned Tom, our senior designer, when Trevor and Donna left the office together for a break.

"Why are they saying they are going to be quick? This is nothing for him to be proud of. I would be ashamed if I were him," said the office junior Tony.

Some mornings, the boys hummed the funny tune from Benny Hill's comedy series together while watching Donna parking her car outside the window. As Donna's car reversed and turned, again and again, the boys sang louder and louder and I laughed.

***

I went to the Royal Ascot races with Trevor's team in June

2017. It was my first race meeting, and I had to buy my first ever fancy hat for that event. I ordered what looked like the hat of my dreams online and kept it in its box until the races. I should have shadowed Donna, who spent lots of time going to shops to try different hats on. In the end she looked stunning while, next to her, I looked like her auntie in my ill-fitting hat, even though I was the slightly younger one.

"Oh no, I look like a clown," I said at first, though my colleagues assured me I looked fine.

Tristan, our foreman, kindly explained how to bet to me. As I reached for some money to make my first bet, Tristan exclaimed, "Ah, I have actually seen your handbag on the inside! Can I have another look? I don't think I have ever seen the inside of a woman's handbag before."

***

"How much have you won so far?" Cameron asked me cheerfully as I phoned him from the races.

"I am anything but winning," I laughed.

Cameron and I had lived together for a few years. He is an outgoing, gregarious joker, but perhaps because he has been through a lot in his life, he also has tons of sensitivity; he has been my rock, my best friend, and my true partner. He is Scottish. After our phone call, I chose to be irrational for a moment, and rather than go for the horses tipped by my well-prepared colleagues, I looked for one whose name would bear some Scottish reference. Having hesitated over a horse called Scottish, I bet on one called Highland Reel. Imagine how surprised I was when I saw Scottish lead the race for most of the time before Highland Reel won the race! I felt this kind of a fluke might not repeat itself. Rather than spend my new money on other races, I treasured it and took it home at the end of the day, for good luck.

"How did you bet? Highland Reel? Did you know about this horse before, or did you just make a random choice?" asked Tristan, who was not used to losing while seeing others win.

The weather was scorching. It was Wednesday: I think it was the third day of the Royal Ascot races in 2017, which had become the hottest day of the year to date. I mostly drank water, partially because I should not drink alcohol while on my medication, but also because I could picture myself tipsy and falling off the stairs in my uncomfortable shoes if I drank any more alcohol in the hot weather. Donna was unlike me. She was a trooper, and she had proper drinks while wearing far higher heels than me. She took plenty of selfies after making all that effort to look great. She succeeded, she looked perfect, and understandably she wanted to capture that.

Trevor generously took the role of my tour guide around different spectator sectors.

"The people above us are the royalty and celebrities," he explained to me, "We are the commoners. But those in the section down there are the peasants."

***

On the last day of my three-month probation period, Trevor asked me to his office to tell me he had decided to extend my probation by another three months.

"I did not like the fact that you used the company funds to buy a new kettle while I was away," he said.

"The kettle broke down. You and Donna were abroad so I could not ask your permission. We had some clients on site who were making their tea with a saucer lying on the kettle top. It was not safe to operate, somebody could get burnt."

In spite of my defence, my probation was extended, and I started looking for a new job again.

CHAPTER TWENTY – KEEP GOING

In 2010, I was prescribed two kinds of medication, an anti-psychotic and an anti-depressant. My prescription has not been changed for more than ten years now. Both those medicines can be dangerous during pregnancy, their respective leaflets warn, and the leaflet attached to my anti-depressant says, 'If you are a woman capable of having children you should use a reliable method of contraception (such as the contraceptive pill) when taking [sertraline].'

Effectively, it seems you are expected to spend your life taking the contraceptive pill if you are a woman on anti-depressants, even if they are prescribing you antidepressants as a precaution, so you don't relapse in future, as in my case. I never started trying for the children that I so much wanted. In 2015 I received a copy of a letter from NHS mental health services with advice to my GP on medication. The letter said, "If there has been more than one episode of psychosis and the patient is stable then it is recommended Ms Weber stay on medication over the long term. If she wants to stop, to do so slowly – […] depending on response."

In reality, no GP of mine ever was interested in monitoring my response and in prescribing me a reduced dose.

"You are ill. You must take your medication," my GPs said emphatically to me.

***

Back in my psychotic days in 2009 Harlesden, a community nurse told me I was going to get better even though I would never be able to lead certain lifestyles.

"Some girls finish their 9 to 5 job, then they work out at the gym, and later in the evening they relax with their boyfriend over a glass of wine," he said. "You will not have this lifestyle. But there are still ways in which you can do well."

Well, Mr Nurse, I nearly got there. Even if wine is missing from my evenings. I have a full-time office job I like. I have a supportive boyfriend I love. I sometimes regret having no children, and we do not own a big house, but I believe that I am living a good life. I only need to avoid mentioning my mental health history outside of this memoir.

**

In early 2021 I received a letter from Post Office Life Insurance inviting me to request a quote for life insurance. Their small print at the back said, "We won't pay a claim on death if it was as a result of suicide or intentional self-inflicted injury […]." I was excited to read this because I hoped this fragment might safeguard them enough to let them offer life insurance to mental health patients like me. I phoned them asking for a quote, adding that I was post-psychotic. Unfortunately, though, I was told that they will not insure a post-psychotic person against an early death.

I also enquired about a life insurance quote for me with Legal & General in early 2021. Their adviser went through their entire health questionnaire with me before turning me down.

"Would it help if I phone again a few months later, after more time has passed?" I asked.

"No, it wouldn't. It's psychosis that was flagged on your application. I can't offer you a quote, I'm sorry," he explained. A post-psychotic person clearly cannot be insured against an early death with Legal & General either.

Although depressed people sometimes feel suicidal, a history of depression does not automatically prevent you from securing yourself some life insurance in this country today. Neither does a history of anxiety. However, a history of psychosis does. It disqualifies you. Most British insurers nowadays assume that a post-psychotic person is not fit for life insurance at any price.

People tend to think a psychotic person is morbid. Yet, I know from my personal experience that psychosis can simply be the name for a spell of extreme anxiety resulting in hallucinations or delusional thinking. Nonetheless, after that spell, you are assigned your label and you are no longer acceptable to some organisations, no matter how stable you return to being. You are forever post-psychotic, and different rules apply to you.

I was lucky. After years of rejections, I had met a good insurance agent who had suggested to me in 2018 that, of all the British insurers, Scottish Widows had seemed the most understanding of mental health problems. We had tried for a policy there, and I had got my life successfully insured.

It is a blessing for me, since being insured is helping me feel less anxious. However, it appears that a few years on, they may still be the only British organisation to insure people like me. Scottish Widows charge me almost precisely twice the monthly premium that Legal & General proposed to me in 2021 for the same amount of cover, before my psychosis was flagged up on their system. It is a relatively expensive insurance, and therefore I sometimes try shopping around for a cheaper option. This is how I keep myself up to date with the market and I know that in early 2021, nearly no British insurers want my custom. To me, this illustrates how little society thinks of people like me.

I am not the only post-psychotic resident of the United Kingdom, and I surely was not the last one to ever break down this way. I would love to leave some positive legacy to younger people by writing about my life. I hope my speaking out may contribute to improving some other people's lives in the future. I would like to let the psychotic woman in the street know that life does not have to always be like that. I would also love to let the insurers know that post-psychotic does not necessarily mean you are dying.

***

After I abruptly stopped taking medication in 2018, I briefly relapsed yet again. I had been feeling lethargic at work, and because my GP did not want to lower my dose, I stopped ordering my tablets altogether, foolishly. I first went through a manic period I think, with my sedative so suddenly absent from my system, although at my new job they simply thought I was very outgoing. My near and dear ones did not pick it up instantly that something was changing. Once faced with some stress at work though, I eventually went through an episode in early 2019. This time they did not register psychosis in my papers, just anxiety, but it was similar to my previous episodes. I posted bizarre messages online. I even tried to message the English royals as well as the Catholic Pope via social media. Fortunately, this time I had my Cameron around. I did not perceive myself as ill, but because I could see Cameron was worried, I let him persuade me he should take me to see the doctor.

I once stood up for hours at night, unable to sleep, too restless to sit down, not wanting to wake Cameron up by fidgeting in the bed next to him. I found some calm and consolation in thinking that, as I stood there, I was guarding our home and his sleep and nothing bad could happen. That lasted until he did wake up and insisted that I should try to lie down. I quickly recovered this time. I was only off work for two months, which gives me an idea of the relative intensity of my episode. My increased social anxiety lingered on as a result.

I got in touch with Paul during my relapse in 2019. He was still in his managerial job and had settled down with his partner. I could see in their Facebook photos that Paul looked so relaxed and happy around her in a way he had never been around me. I wrote to tell him that. It was nice exchanging a few messages after so many years, though neither of us feels the need to continue keeping in touch. I was relieved he was fine, and I got some closure.

After I messaged him on LinkedIn, Nathan Meadowbank wrote back to me very politely to say he wished me well, but he also wrote that he remembered nothing and no-one from Clever Costs. I replied that this was because there had been nothing for him to remember, as nobody beside him had been saying anything much. Naturally, I am sure that since he now has high-profile function at his workplace, he chooses not to remember. It would be unusual for anyone to remember "nothing and no-one" from a workplace they had spent years at.

I researched a few other people and companies I have mentioned in this memoir.

Eddie built a good career in some exciting corporations, which I learnt without contacting him.

Five Stars went bust.

Clever Costs was bought by an international fintech giant for millions of pounds, and they no longer have a London office.

As I mentioned before, the surgery I had worked for was closed down.

Jeff was declared bankrupt after losing his career as a doctor.

I still feel happiest in the background of businesses, in the relatively invisible supporting roles. However, my supporting roles have evolved in terms of responsibility and remuneration, and I now feel entirely satisfied with my post-psychotic career path. I have eventually got myself a corporate job, too. On my health side, in 2022, I was diagnosed with cancer. I know I could possibly die soon. It is not an easy experience for me, but, for now, I prefer my current experience of early cancer to my former experience of acute psychosis. Unlike the way I felt during my psychosis, during my cancer I am not ashamed of being ill. Everything around me is understandable, and everyone is being incredibly nice to me.

Cameron stands by my side. He continues to be my rock to lean on and my comforter to laugh with. Thus, I have found my big love after all, and this time I know for sure this is "it." If I live long enough, I would love to write more about Cameron in another book.

***

We all went through months of lockdown due to the Covid-19 pandemic in the UK in 2020. Anxiety and depression are said to be rife following the pandemic. I do not know about the statistics for other mental health conditions. I know for a fact though that there is always a light at the end of the tunnel for those who are struggling with their mental health. All you need to do is keep going. Never doubt it. You truly can get better with time. As the sun rises again, and again, the new days will softly kiss your healing wounds like fresh sterile dressings.

Milton Keynes UK
Ingram Content Group UK Ltd.
UKHW021858231124
451423UK00005B/462

9 781835 634714